# PRAISE FOR *GRAVITY &*

"In my years of being a musician, I've learned that music is the sound of feelings; and as a yogi, I've learned that yoga is the way emotions feel in my body. *Gravity & Grace* encourages us to unlock those feelings, let them come to the surface, sit with them, breathe them, and let go of the expectations we have about them so that they may pass. This is an inspiring read for yogis who've practiced for decades and those who are just beginning their journeys on the mat."
                                        **MICHAEL FRANTI**
                                        musician, filmmaker, and activist

"Terrific yoga books, like terrific teachers, reveal ourselves to ourselves. In his profoundly intuitive book, Peter can connect to every reader as easily as he can connect to each student in a yoga class. *Gravity & Grace* is like having a teacher by your side."
                                        **MICHELLE JACOBI**
                                        founder of Centre de Yoga du Marais (Paris, France);
                                        professor of yoga, University of South Florida

"*Gravity & Grace* should be required reading, unquestionably, for all yoga teachers and dedicated practitioners, but more surprisingly to me, for anyone keenly interested in living a happier life. Peter brilliantly illuminates how the conscious movement of our physical body influences our state of being, and therefore ultimately, our mental health and happiness. The book itself is a master yoga class. It changed me."
                                        **BLAKE BELTRAM**
                                        cofounder of MINDBODY

"I loved this book. Peter has written a rare personal story of his own journey—one filled with hard-won insights woven around some serious study and modern research that makes the art and science of yoga very accessible. In this day and age of physical, fitness-based yoga, this is a refreshing change, and any student interested in the healing gifts that yoga promises through awakening the subtle body will find plenty of helpful and inspiring ideas here."
                                        **GUNNAR LOVELACE**
                                        founder of ThriveMarket.com

"*Gravity & Grace* is both a fitting title for Peter Sterios's long-awaited book, as well as a description of his fluid approach to yoga. He fully embodies the grounding nature of gravity as well as the lightness of grace in how he approaches his personal practice, the clarity and understanding in his teaching, his presence, and his thoughtful words. Peter's conversational book explores what it really means to be a practicing yogi in the modern world. It is a must-read—one that explores the central theme of just how we practice, as well as how we navigate the core questions of life. Buy this book and give in. Send it to all of your friends. Read it again and again and listen for the nuances of meaning found within."

FELICIA TOMASKO
editor-in-chief of *LA Yoga* and *BOSTON Yoga*;
president of Bliss Network

"Peter is a master in questioning all the rules and pushing the boundaries of how we understand yoga. In *Gravity & Grace*, he reorients us towards a more present, embodied relationship to yoga. His words instruct us how to develop grounded curiosity in relationship to our bodies, movement, and intuitive wisdom. His stories speak to the profound potential that yoga has to transform and integrate. His experience inspires us to revel in the intersections between science and spirituality. If you are looking for a new perspective on intimacy, in life, and with yoga, this book is for you."

KATIE CLANCY
founder of Soma Yoga (Durango, CO); writer

"Peter's work, and his delightful book *Gravity & Grace*, expresses something more—beyond what the modern yoga collective has absorbed—which lights a way for yogis new and old to deeply explore the mysterious hidden quality of yoga that has clearly shaped his life into something magical! This culminating work is obviously not a beginning for him, and yet it is! Where he is headed, only God knows, but he is in league with the Masters that came before him. He will certainly be a beacon for humanity while shedding clarity and light on a path that leads us hOMe."

MARC AND HEATHER TITUS
co-creators of Sedona Yoga Festival

"Perhaps the truest yoga is simply and purely being with the ground of what is. In revealing his own process and journey, Peter honestly and humbly invites us on the path to uncover the perennial wisdoms abiding in our own stories and bodies as medicine or empowerment for awakening. Integrating science, physiology, the mat, and the cushion, *Gravity & Grace* masterfully reveals a method and impeccable way of transcending the habitual perceptions in our practice, on the mat and beyond, to taste the authentic fruit of yoga."    **DR. ROBERT B. NORETT, DC**
founder of Stillpoint Health Center (Los Angeles, CA);
board certification in Integrative Medicine

"Brilliant! In Peter Sterios's new book *Gravity & Grace*, he provides clear, beautifully written insights for creating a deeply personal yoga practice. Beyond that, this book helps the reader move into a more integrated, connected life. Whether you are a beginner or an experienced yogi, *Gravity & Grace* provides a profound path with sure-footed guidance. I recommend it highly."    **ERIK OLESEN**
licensed psychotherapist; certified Neurofeedback trainer;
author of *Mastering the Winds of Change*

"Finally! A how-to-practice yoga book that has nothing to do with putting the body into required shapes and everything to do with understanding the metaphysical aspects of practice through a practical, scientific lens. Peter shares rich stories from his many decades of practice and teaching that illuminate the subtle nature and power of yoga, and make it SO easy for any practitioner to explore and play with his suggested principles of practice on their mat. *Gravity & Grace* is a must-have reference for any yoga practitioner or teacher. I LOVE this book!"    **KARA-LEAH GRANT**
author of *Forty Days of Yoga* and
*Sex, Drugs & (Mostly) Yoga*

"*Gravity & Grace* sums up Peter Sterios's yoga journey for me in one word: trailblazer. As you read his book, I think there's one thing we can all agree on—you can't fake gravity, physically or emotionally. How Peter has overcome adversity through yoga is empowering and inspiring. If you're early in your practice or someone who has been doing yoga for decades, *Gravity & Grace* is a must-read for your practice, and way, way beyond it."

DIAMOND DALLAS PAGE
author of *Positively Unstoppable: The Art of Owning It*;
founder of DDP Yoga; former Heavyweight Champion
Wrestler/WWE Hall of Fame (2017)

"My first experience of Peter's teaching at a conference was enchanting through his verbal precision with every cue and the subtle nature of what I experienced from pose to pose. It is no surprise to feel that same quality in his book *Gravity & Grace*. He offers a refreshing new outlook to practicing asana and helps restore the creativity that lives within each of us without forgetting the yoga that got us to where we are. He has found a way to articulate his stories and experiences with intellectual prowess made simple. Peter truly empowers students and teachers alike to trust themselves and paves a realistic path to help us discover and connect with our inner subtle guides. Be ready to break old thinking about westernized yoga and get ready to feel something truly soulful."

JOHN SALISBURY
founder of Modern Yoga (Scottsdale, AZ)

"When Peter's 20-year apprenticeship with his long-time teacher ended abruptly, he was sent out into the yoga world figuratively as naked as a newborn baby. With this book, we see how—after many years of intense study, self-investigation, and creative experimentation—he's grown into a full-fledged yoga adult. *Gravity & Grace* is both an inspiration for all aspiring 'inner' teachers and a remarkable education in the subtle dimension for any teacher from any yoga school, no matter how many years of experience."

RICHARD ROSEN
author of *Yoga FAQ, Original Yoga,*
and *The Yoga of Breath*

"I'm so excited to finally have this long-awaited book in my hands—to hold, to highlight, to earmark pages, and to refer to as a manual for life on and off my mat. It's a brilliant guide that is also an amazing read (and re-read) for anyone looking to delve within the divine heart space of yoga. *Gravity & Grace* is more than just an incredible journey in the subtle nuances of the heArt of Yoga. This book is a memoir, a primer, a secret source, and a truly cherished gift! Thank you, Peter!"                   **HELENA ZERA, RN**
                              foundress of Vyana Yoga (Manlius, NY)
                              and Hastapada®

"This book is an excellent read for beginners and advanced students alike. It presents new and fresh research to back ancient tradition and practices. Peter is clearly a master teacher for a reason. After 40 years of personal practice, he lays out a solid foundation for how he came to the concepts of gravity, grace, and levity, and how to practice them. His story is touching and the practices are deeply insightful. I loved learning the minute details of how to achieve space in the body through the subtle layers, and I have been practicing his techniques each day. A nagging hamstring injury has all but disappeared in just a week, and I even went for a run this morning, which I haven't done in years! We really do have the power to heal ourselves through yoga and the subtle layers of prana."                   **ASHLEY MELIN**
                              founder of SoulJour (Portland, OR)

"Peter's insights provide a fresh lens for the complex and often contradictory wild world of yoga. His journey to discover how yoga teaches us integrates modern science with traditional yogic philosophy and remarkable insights from his many years of studying with some of yoga's greatest innovators. His approach is the next evolution of this empowering practice—finding the deep connection to one another and uncovering inner peace and joy. *Gravity & Grace* is a book I will go back to again and again."

                              **WENDY KLEIN**
                              founder of Nandi Yoga (San Mateo, CA)

"Through his first book, Peter Sterios beautifully elucidates the divine connection of gravity and grace in simple language. The clarity in his writing helps show you how to apply these two terms in the practice of yoga and other life processes. Our body is a composite of the finite and the infinite. Peter shows clearly how that realization can be uncovered. I highly recommend this heartful book for all students of yoga."

MALAV DANI
founder of meFree (Mumbai, India)

"Through Peter's first book, *Gravity & Grace*, I feel like I've journeyed through the mysterious energetic cave of ancient yoga and found the hidden treasure that very few modern teachers are able to express with such profound clarity. His lifetime dedication and authenticity in yoga shine through as he shares the subtle body gifts yoga promises and his articulate teaching so effectively delivers. This is a book I will return to, and often."

MASOOD ALI KHAN, PHD
energy medicine teacher; musician; actor; model

"Sitting down to read and absorb the insights found in *Gravity & Grace* was an absolute joy. Peter is one of my guiding teachers of yoga, and I felt the very essence of his teaching transmitted on each page. The book, like his classes, takes the reader on a powerful journey, carefully and seamlessly weaving the threads between the physical body, subtle anatomy, philosophy, story, and asana to create a rich tapestry of wisdom that envelops you. I have practiced for over 20 years and still learned so much from Peter's rich writing. I will be including this book as essential reading in all of my future teacher trainings, which I am sure will inspire teachers and all students of yoga for many years to come."

NIKKI RALSTON
founder of Urban Ashram studios (Auckland, New Zealand); creator of The Ralston Method

"What an amazing journey this book created for me. I felt like I was being held by divine grace with every page. I experienced healing, a deep exhale, just reading the book. I can only imagine the healing and growth that will come from putting what I learned here into practice."

AMY PUNZEL, LTCOL
USMC (Jacksonville, NC)

"*Gravity & Grace* is a brilliant new 'light' on yoga. Peter Sterios combines eloquent stories from his 40-plus years of practice and direct learning from some of the most renowned yoga masters in the world—with meticulous scientific research to offer a fluid and intuitive style of Hatha yoga accessible to all. He invites those of us trained in rigorous, exacting yoga styles to reconsider our practice, much like life, as a journey where each pose offers an opportunity to explore and burnish the hard edges of our physical, mental, and emotional states. The main thesis of the book revolves around the point that the real teacher is within our subconscious. Peter's book is a blueprint for us to find that real teacher within, and to take our practice and experience of life to the next level."     **RAMIN HEYDARPOUR**
founder of FLEX R&D

"Peter Sterios's new book is a wonderful synthesis of his two professions. In many ways, he has developed an original architectural integration of the structure of the mind and body in yoga. He guides readers through their own unique personal voyage of self-discovery, physically and psychologically, by employing our nature's finest gifts of gravity and grace."

**ERNEST AND KATHRYN ROSSI, PHD**
authors of *The Collected Works of Milton H. Erickson, MD*

"Peter Sterios so emulates what he teaches in his book *Gravity & Grace*. From the very first moment we met, his grace was palpable. For him to piece together the abstract qualities of the subtle body, and to describe them in a way that can be understood and also benefit even the newest student of yoga, is a testimony of his skills and genuine talent. Thank you, Peter. Your book is a gift."     **RINA JAKUBOWICZ**
author of *The Yoga Mind: 52 Essential Principles
of Yoga Philosophy to Deepen Your Practice*

# GRAVITY
## grace

# GRAVITY & *grace*

*How to Awaken*

*Your Subtle Body*

*and the Healing*

*Power of Yoga*

## PETER STERIOS

FOREWORD BY EOIN FINN

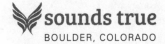

**sounds true**
BOULDER, COLORADO

Sounds True
Boulder, CO 80306

This book is not intended as a substitute for the medical recommendations of
physicians or other health-care providers. Rather, it is intended to offer information
to help the reader cooperate with physicians and health-care providers in a mutual
quest for optimal well-being. We advise readers to carefully review and understand
the ideas presented and to seek the advice of a qualified professional before
attempting to use them.

Published 2019

Cover design by Tara DeAngelis
Book design by Beth Skelley
Illustrations © 2019 Kara Fellows

Cover photo © Mikki Willis, ELEVATE Films

Grateful acknowledgment is made to Three Leaves Press/Doubleday for permission
to reprint excerpts from Michael Roach and Christie McNally's *The Essential Yoga
Sutra: Ancient Wisdom for Your Yoga*.

Printed in Canada

Library of Congress Cataloging-in-Publication Data

Names: Sterios, Peter, author.
Title: Gravity and grace : how to awaken your subtle body and the healing
    power of yoga / Peter Sterios.
Description: Boulder, CO : Sounds True, 2019. | Includes bibliographical
    references. | Summary: "Mastering the subtle body for maximum healing
    with yoga"—Provided by publisher.
Identifiers: LCCN 2018058281 (print) | LCCN 2019980910 (ebook) |
    ISBN 9781683641810 (paperback) | ISBN 9781683642039 (ebook)
Subjects: LCSH: Hatha yoga. | Healing.
Classification: LCC RA781.7 .S7279 2019 (print) | LCC RA781.7 (ebook) |
    DDC 613.7/046—dc23
LC record available at https://lccn.loc.gov/2018058281
LC ebook record available at https://lccn.loc.gov/2019980910

10 9 8 7 6 5 4 3 2 1

To the people, teachers, and students who
have influenced my life in a way no book,
video, or podcast ever could—with presence.

Grace fills empty spaces, but it can only
enter where there is a void to receive it,
and it is grace itself which makes this void.

**Simone Weil**

# Contents

# Foreword

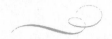

We use the word *alignment* all the time to describe yoga poses, but when two human minds are aligned, it is pure magic.

When I first got to know Peter, we had both just finished teaching yoga at a five-day festival in the Bali highlands of Ubud. I loved the people and the energy there, but I do remember the utter relief in my body at the prospect of heading down to the coast at the festival's end. There was nothing I wanted to do more than hurl myself into the steep, barreling ocean waves Indonesia is famed for. Peter and I shared a taxi to where we were both staying in the coastal town of Canggu, Bali, and immediately began talking about our respective yoga journeys and philosophies. It was a conversation that began at the start of a two-hour drive through the thick Bali traffic and went on for days. Though the ocean was calling me, I couldn't leave the cafe we were sitting in. Peter and I talked the whole day. We were hanging off each other's words, excited that the discoveries we held so dear were shared by another teacher.

I'm thrilled to see that so much of what lit me up in those conversations is now presented in this book. *Gravity & Grace* is precisely the direction in which modern yoga needs to move. There are plenty of books that teach the technique of each *asana*: "Move the ribs this way; make the leg straight." But learning the language of the subtle body so that yoga is no longer one size fits all, but instead unique to the needs of *every* body, is something that yoga practitioners are thirsting for. Even the ones who don't yet know they are thirsting for it will be when they read these insights.

*Gravity & Grace* is a return to the roots of *hatha* yoga. When you read classical yoga texts such as the *Hatha Yoga Pradipika*, it is obvious that the original yogis were not concerned so much about achieving some kind of perfect shape in the pose; yoga was nothing close to the gymnastics competition that we have allowed it to become. What mattered was the internal experience of each yoga practitioner. Yogis were focused on the energy flow in the body. They were concerned about cultivating maximum health and vitality so their individual energies could be more in harmony with the universe.

As much as *Gravity & Grace* is a return to this original intention, it is also an incredible progression. Peter's work is respectful to lineage and makes the map of the subtle body the yogis left us easy to understand. But there is not a lot written in the ancient yogic texts about how we can work with those maps. Peter has used his own explorations of the inner workings of yoga, a mindful awareness of bodily sensations, and cutting-edge science to create the definitive guide to the territory.

Your concept of what constitutes "advanced yoga" will shift dramatically through Peter's work. Advanced yoga, to most people, is about reaching some kind of perfect expression of a complex pose. But advanced yoga is really about tuning in to the inner teacher. I call this teacher *the wise guide inside*; Peter calls it *the teacher within*.

In yoga and in almost all aspects of modern living, we have lost the ability to listen to the wisdom of our bodies; instead, we seek the approval of others as the source of our happiness. As Peter points out in this book, one of the basic questions people need to stop asking is, "Am I doing this pose *right*?" Instead we need to tune in to the "rightness" of the pose by how it *feels*.

I completely share this viewpoint. In my own work, I describe it this way: yoga is a feeling, not a shape. The instant we make the shape of the pose more important than the feeling of calm, grounded centeredness, the practice risks becoming yet another rat race. As soon as we start looking at the poses in terms of aesthetic perfection, we are working from the outside in. We start forcing our bodies into shapes using our will and muscular effort without listening and feeling whether it is good for us. All too often in yoga, we end up sticking square pegs into round holes.

We have inherited a uniform concept of the perfect pose, but *Gravity & Grace* makes clear that each of us has different blocks that need to be addressed in each pose. Some of these blocks are physical, and some exist deep in our psychology. The biggest joy in yoga *asana* is about releasing these areas. So much freedom emerges when we do this.

The problem has been this: even if yoga practitioners want to access their inner wisdom to let it guide them through the poses, until the release of *Gravity & Grace*, there had not been a book that explains exactly *how*. This book intelligently maps out the process. We benefit not just from the four decades Peter has on the mat but also from the way his mind works. It is not often we get such a perfect synergy of right- and left-brain thinking. This work was created by someone who understands how to express the process of listening and guiding the body from the inside out from both a rational point of view and the artistic, feeling experience—it is a rare fusion. This is what makes Peter such a great teacher and *Gravity & Grace* so powerful. Besides yoga, Peter's other career and passion is architecture. Like good architecture, a good yoga pose should allow us to feel expansive and connected to the outer world and not trapped inside our own walls. It is about creating spaces that flow—and ultimately ones that let in light.

*Gravity & Grace* is not just the same old, same old. This book turns the practice of yoga from art into science so we can understand it—and then back into art again so it doesn't become dry. It does this masterfully, and it is a joy to read. It is not a recipe book for techniques of how to do a pose. Instead, it is an elegant distillation of practical principles that can be applied to one's own unique experience. In a yoga pose, as with life, can we create flow where once there was resistance? Can we soften into where there is resistance instead of fighting it so much?

The stories Peter tells about how this process was revealed to him are insightful, real, and moving. Yoga poses and life both make us confront uncomfortable edges. Loss and challenge can be our greatest teachers, if we let them. One of the losses we learn about is when Peter's "core-teacher," Shandor Remete, a man who deeply inspired his journey, abruptly ended their teacher-student relationship. After twenty years of training, being unexpectedly cut loose set Peter into a tailspin, but it also paved the way for him to experience the practice of yoga in the refined way we learn about in *Gravity & Grace*. Other doors, too, seem to close: there is a health issue and then a back injury, things that could be devastating to a yoga teacher's career. Instead, all of these events became the proverbial invisible hand guiding Peter toward what this book is essentially about: preparing students for "the ultimate solo journey—toward the inner teacher we all embody" that awakens the tools to listen more to their own subtle body.

All too often, Peter reminds us, we want to dominate our bodies with our busy minds. Our mind becomes the captain of the ship shouting orders at the body, not listening to the needs of the body or the language of sensation it speaks. The poses are something we *do*, but we don't *feel*. Yet injuries force us to listen. They are invitations to show up for our own selves and correct the imbalances in our relationships with our own bodies. These skills, in turn, allow us to heal the relationships with others in our lives. To do this, we need to slow down and shift from doing to being. When we get really good at listening and being instead of forcing, we call it "well-being."

The breath is a great place to start, and Peter's book makes the powerful effects of the breath accessible. How to breathe is simple; we do it all day. But how to breathe well is a skill. Like playing an instrument, it needs to be learned and practiced. Few yoga books are as insightful as Peter's for unpacking the process of breathing as a way of accessing our internal guidance system in order to make the poses more sustainable.

Likewise, the principles he introduces for *asana* are simple yet sophisticated. Albert Einstein has been quoted as saying, "Everything should be as simple as it can be, but not simpler." *Gravity & Grace* is a testament to this statement. The principles outlined are elegant and profoundly impactful. They are easy to understand, and each one brings more ease, flow, and grace into our experience on and off the mat.

Gravity is the force in the universe that keeps all physical objects connected. Grace is its spiritual equivalent. Here's wishing you, the reader, receptivity to these incredible forces in your journey. May you live feeling their pull on your orbit and their blessings forever awakened in your heart.

**Eoin Finn**

Yogi, author, teacher, surfer,
and founder of Blissology

# Preface

Consciously, the writing of this book began twelve years ago, although I sense it started much earlier. As with most creative impulses, determining when and where the seeds for a book originate is mysterious. What first showed up for me was faint and rather unassuming; it appeared now and then as a soft inner voice, noticeably at moments of deep concentration or stillness, that gently disrupted my practice with something like, "Hey, friend, pay attention. This would be helpful to share with students." It was a different, unfamiliar kind of voice, quiet and subtle—not the noisy, mostly selfish "me" chatter of the busy life I was leading at the time. Initially, these small intrusions were easy to remember, allowing practice to continue with total recall. Over time, however, they became increasingly detailed and complex—and more frequent. Five journals filled with notes were the result—much of it in a cryptic, unstructured form of writing.

What follows is a story drawn from those roughly two years' worth of musings that a calm voice within provided during practice, interwoven with personal observations of the yoga I have lived for forty-plus years of teaching and studying. I also share how experiences on and off the mat helped refine my ability to see and hear what lay obscured in my writing, my teaching, and my life, and to feel the presence of miracles happening all along.

The real reasons I wrote this book became clear once the writing was finished. Up to that point, the question of "why" had seemed irrelevant, since I didn't know when I started writing where it would lead. First off, the pages that await you are the result of a calling to write, figuratively and literally—first, as practice notes, and much later, as a book. Although it took over ten years to realize the full extent of the "call," I now view this gestation period as perfect timing that naturally allowed life to provide what I needed to see clearly: that in my notes from unexpected lessons on my mat lay something worthwhile, though unfinished.

Just as the fresh outlook that time had provided was renewing my motivation to decipher and expand my original notes, an email appeared from an editor at Sounds True, inquiring whether I would consider writing a book based on my upcoming yoga retreat at Esalen Institute in Big Sur, California, a magical place where I've been able to explore the edges of modern yoga in direct interaction with students from around the world. The retreat's workshop, called "Gravity and Grace: Tools for Rewiring the Subtle Body," incorporated the principles of yoga that I have used and taught for the past twenty years and that form the essence of this book. In a mysterious way, the email sent a clear message, unknown to the sender, reminding me that, truly, "miracles are nature unimpeded."[1] The coincidental connection of events was there to support and strengthen my desire to write afresh—to take numerous journals full of notes and tales and transform them into a book. It also helped me trust that uncovering and sharing stories from my practice and life could be beneficial to others, even people I may never meet.

I have approached the writing of this book as a nonmystical attempt to describe the mystical healing powers found in the practice of yoga, particularly those of the subtle body, using simple language and personal analogies. My desire is to provide an accessible learning perspective for any student, at any level, practicing any style of yoga, so they may see for themselves the wonders of gravity and grace that have revealed themselves to me.

Training is believing what you are told.
Education is remembering what you know.

**Charles L. Moore**

# *Introduction*

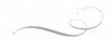

From its start millennia ago to the present, the path of yoga is often traveled by those with a passionate desire to learn more about themselves and life. Usually it begins with simple body exercises that create a new awareness, arising first on a physical level. Then, through consistent practice, the magic and mystery of yoga unfold the potential to transform on levels beyond the physical—into the psychological and, even further, into the spiritual.

Somewhere along our life journey, the seed of yoga is planted by an encounter with someone or something—a casual meeting with a teacher, a friend who practices, or a video or article; it then germinates into the action of doing yoga. With action comes experience that is received through one or more of our five senses. This activates perception, and we identify and label the experience, usually as positive or negative. In turn, this perception inevitably creates insight, emotion, and energy, which support either continuing yoga practice to seek more of the experience or ceasing practice to avoid it. Because you are reading this, it's safe to say that at this moment, the yoga seed within you supports your practice with enough potency to arouse curiosity and lead you further.

This could be the perfect moment for *Gravity & Grace* to come your way. Drawing on my experience and perspective as a yoga practitioner who has met himself on the mat each day for some forty-five years and as a yoga teacher who has taught thousands of classes and workshops, I wrote this book to lend added dimension to the next leg of your yoga journey, a new perspective with the potential to transform your practice. Here you will not find advocacy for any particular yoga style or tradition. This is not a how-to manual instructing you in how to shape your body into the ideal pose in the ideal way. While it does offer instruction centered on common poses (*asana*), this instruction is less about how to *do* the pose and more about how to *be* the pose, engaging all levels of yourself—physical, mental, and spiritual—and both of your yoga bodies—the physiology of flesh and bone and the movement of subtle energy. In fact, this book aims to teach you how to let yourself be *guided by* subtle energy as you move on your mat.

Many years of study with the influential yoga teachers of my life led me to want to create a method of practice that would allow a unique expression of movement while recognizing the personal limitations each one of us comes to yoga with. The challenge was to discover a way to practice that empowers each individual to find the path to the pure potential of their unique physical form and to build the mental awareness necessary for self-healing and restoring balance in their lives.

To achieve this, the first task is to awaken in the practitioner the self-authority for creating movement safely and efficiently in each practice. Then, with their own personal experience as a guide, the next task is to build intuitive motivation for going further and deeper into the subtle body aspects of their practice.

To this end, the goal of the guidance found in this book is to minimize mental distraction with technique and intuitively focus attention on experiencing the essence and beauty of movement and the sensations produced during practice. Thus, we access the transformative grace of a practice tuned to present-moment experience and learn to use the natural gift of subtle energies that we are all born with in service of our growth and healing. This is the terrain you are about to enter.

## A TOUR OF THE BOOK

To start acquainting you with the underlying principles in this approach, in part 1, "Teaching Stories," I take you into the key experiences that led me to discover them. The first chapters contain teaching stories from my own yoga journey to give you an understanding of the origins of the approach and to show how they emerged in real life. Part 2, "The Energies of Gravity and Grace," delves into the mysteries of subtle energies conceptually, with a discussion of gravity and grace lending new perspective for your journey forward.

In part 3, "Science and Yoga Meet," we'll explore the nature of the human body that we all bring to our yoga practice, both its *gravity* dimension—in this sense of the word, meaning the known, three-dimensional anatomical and physiologic systems—and the *grace* that operates in parallel—that is, the subtle realms that recent science is now uncovering. Here you'll find perspectives from emerging sciences on some of the truths about the body-mind that the ancient yogis knew and used in designing the practices of yoga.

Part 4, "Subtle Body Anatomy," introduces the main contours of the vessels and systems that move subtle energy through the body: the *chakras*, *nadis*, *bhutas*, *vayus*, and *marmas*. And finally, in part 5, "Practice Essentials," it will be time for you to practice. Here I teach you how to cultivate awareness of the flow of subtle body energy in common poses on your mat, and I share key principles that apply in any yoga pose (*asana*). When you incorporate these principles into your regular practice, your sensitivity to subtle body forces will naturally increase and strengthen your relationship to the life force you're born with. My hope is that it will deepen your experience of yoga—and of life.

# PART 1

## *Teaching Stories*

The principles I offer in this book are the product of decades of exploring yoga and the subtle body, and thousands upon thousands of hours spent on the mat. They are also inextricably linked to pivotal experiences on my yoga journey. At first, some of these experiences appeared disastrous, generating much pain and suffering in me, physically and emotionally. Ultimately, though, hindsight has taught me that they were portals of discovery. These unexpected stumbles led to insights that profoundly transformed my yoga practice—and my life—and they continue to guide my work as a yoga teacher today. So, let me share with you now some stories about the evolution of gravity and grace as they appeared to me, on and off the mat.

I am the teacher of athletes,
He that by me spreads a wider breast
than my own proves the width of my own,
He most honors my style who learns
under it to destroy the teacher.

**Walt Whitman**

# 1

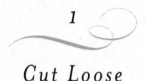

## Cut Loose

Yoga has many traditional adages. One of the best known is, "When the student is ready, the teacher appears." This was so true for me. In the early 1970s, there were few yoga studios in the United States and none where I lived. With internet search engines still decades away, finding a class required effort and luck. Most classes were inconspicuously located in whatever low-cost venues pioneer teachers of yoga could afford: cluttered senior centers, unkempt municipal halls, or, in my case, a windowless, fluorescent-lit space at a university fitness center adjacent to a noisy weight room. My relationship with yoga then was casual, and my practice was often a token effort, unfashionably ahead of its time, done before a workout.

That changed when I moved overseas and met the teacher my yoga path had in store for me, Shandor Remete. I knew very little about the myriad traditions of yoga, but it was clear to me after one workshop that I had found a teacher—a master, actually—who I would end up studying with for the next twenty years. I became dedicated to following him and only him, something rare in today's world of "convenient yoga." He was old school, with a charismatic and at times fierce presence that I respected. At the time, I felt like I was one of few men doing yoga, and I had never met a male yoga teacher; so meeting him was a refreshing change. He was an athlete, as was I, and I appreciated the language he used. He had an uncanny ability to articulate new ways in which my stiff, male body and linear mentality could move, taking me beyond the limited understanding I had of myself.

With Shandor, I became a master of following, as I understood apprenticeship to be a time-honored rite for students of one of the most respected yoga lineages of India, the Iyengar method. I spent many hours a day practicing what he taught me, doing everything he instructed me to do. My proficiency and skill in following, combined with a body type and mental disposition that resembled many of the teachers in that lineage, gave me special status in the yoga community I was becoming a part of. Gaining that status became a built-in reward system that perpetuated even more following on my part; eventually, this earned me the role of assisting Shandor during his trainings and handling many of the administrative tasks for his North American tours. And when a busy international teaching schedule didn't allow him to fulfill all the invitations he received, I became a stand-in, taking his place in studios he didn't have time to get to.

As my reputation spread, I received more invitations to teach—something Shandor encouraged—at studios that wanted a lighter version of his style taught by someone a little less intense. In this way, I became his top American ambassador during those years. I felt privileged that he was part of my life and grateful for the strong personal connection between us. It seemed everything was as it should be and I was "on the path."

And then, without my noticing exactly how it happened, my long apprenticeship was over. It was an abrupt and unpleasant surprise. In hindsight, I could have seen the signs had I paid more attention.

What was to be my last year with Shandor started with slight feelings of impatience and a longing to learn and experience some of the special practices (*kriyas*) he did when we practiced together privately; these *kriyas* cultivated the mystical powers (*siddhis*) he occasionally spoke about. I had read amazing stories in old yoga texts about these esoteric practices, and I assumed that instruction in them was something only advanced and sincere students "earned" the right to receive.

What I didn't understand then was that I lacked certain prerequisites. It wasn't until years later that I could clearly see the most important prerequisite I had not yet attained: overcoming the limitations of being a "follower." Moving to the next level of any truly important endeavor requires getting rid of some things accumulated along the way—things that may have served their purpose in the moment but will be of little or no use in moving forward—and accepting this as it should be. Being someone else's apprentice was something I had to leave behind.

On the last day of the life I had known with my "guru," he asked me to take a short walk with him. Two months earlier I had left him a long voice message—too long, really, to convey what was essentially a request that we discuss the possibility of his teaching me the practices I felt ready to receive. This prompted what I heard as a hopeful message in reply: "Sure, it's time we talk." Now, after a month of traveling and assisting him with his programs without his mentioning this talk, he was about to catch a flight home to Australia. The window for conversation was short.

As we walked in silence, I had a sense something big was about to happen. We arrived at a small park in the neighborhood where I lived and sat quietly on a bench under the shade of an old, twisted oak, watching kids running around being kids. As I waited for him to speak, every part of me was anticipating expressions of appreciation for my years of service, maybe even a little recognition as one of his top students, and *finally*, his approval to learn what was reserved for those in my position. After several minutes, he broke the silence.

"Peter, there are two things in life you never want to be—a soldier or an apprentice."

His words were a shock, even as their full meaning escaped me at first. My body felt numb. My mind flooded with thoughts as I tried to understand how that statement applied to me.

Shandor turned to me, well aware of the turmoil raging inside, and his next, unforgettable—though not uncharacteristic—words were simply, "It's time to get off the tit."

After two decades of devotion to the teacher, just like that, it was over.

We walked back to my house without speaking; the closeness we had shared for years was replaced by a cold, businesslike formality.

The taxi arrived for his ride to the airport, and he walked through my front door without a word of goodbye. I stepped onto the porch and watched him approach the cab. Unexpectedly, he paused and turned back toward me. *Is he having a change of heart?* I wondered.

"Oh, by the way, please don't teach anything I ever taught you" were his parting words.

## ESCAPE TO INDIA

In the period that followed, my confusion was crippling. Many things in my personal and professional life unraveled. I stopped teaching yoga; I had no idea what to teach. Depression was a frequent companion, and practicing yoga didn't help, especially "his" yoga—so I stopped that, too. Months passed. My health deteriorated, and my body ached. Many of the physical conditions yoga had helped me overcome surfaced again, and a new, more serious affliction came up during a routine physical. Clearly, every aspect of my life was out of balance. I sought help from Western and alternative medical doctors but got nowhere.

Then, at the recommendation of a friend, I put my life on hold and traveled to southern India to spend ten weeks at an Ayurvedic hospital for a holistic medical treatment program (*panchakarma*) to reset balance in my life, both physically and psychologically.

## A VISIT FROM HANUMAN

During the first two weeks in India, the medical condition I had been diagnosed with worsened. I felt like I was completely losing control, and a deep despair lurked everywhere my thoughts carried me. I had inescapable feelings of hopelessness—there was nothing I could *do* to help myself.

Then one hot, sleepless night, in a room dimly lit by the other-worldly orange tint of a streetlight, I lay in bed under a mosquito net, considering my own death—*this could be the last night of my life.*

At some point, I drifted into a restless sleep and dreamed. In the dream, I was aware of watching my body asleep on the hospital bed, uncovered and naked. I noticed—and it somehow seemed funny to me—that my arms had become extremely hairy, like those of a gorilla; my hands rested gently on my chest; and my fingertips were oddly positioned along the edges of my breastbone, aligned with my heart. Through my past studies of Indian mythology, I knew of the Hindu deity Hanuman, the monkey-headed man/god often portrayed in artistic renditions ripping open his rib cage to expose his beating heart. However, this image did not come immediately to mind—until, in the dream, my fingernails began digging through the skin into the costal facets of my sternum, clawing at the cartilage that secured my ribs to the bone. The witnessing presence in my dream suddenly became anxious, fearing the sight of a soon-to-be exposed heart; it desperately wanted to escape, to wake up out of the dream.

Simultaneously, in what was now a semi-lucid state, I felt a slight tickle on my chest. Curious, I lifted my head to see the face of a monstrous cockroach staring back at me. In a panic, I sat up and slapped the bug off me. I was wide awake and had an angry, flying pest trapped inside the mosquito net, buzzing my head. My heart was pumping, and I was possessed by a maniacal rage to kill. I jumped to my feet, trapped the roach in the net, and crushed it with my bare hands.

As I stood trembling beside my bed with triggers of fear still firing in my nervous system, a heavy wave of despair crashed over me. So alone in that moment, I was ready to die. I lay down on the bare concrete floor, flat on my back, arms and legs spread-eagle, and begged whatever god there was to take me, to end this life that was no longer worth living.

The swarm of mosquitos that turned up nightly descended onto my exposed body in a feeding frenzy. I didn't care; I didn't move. With no urge to resist, I felt each bite. I thought, *If this is the way God is taking me, devoured by mosquitos, so be it,* and I found the thought strangely comforting. Miraculously, I then fell into a deep sleep.

In the morning, I awoke slowly, unsure of where I was, with sunlight streaming across my face. Still lying flat on my back, I noticed an unusual inner calm. I had slept for hours on a concrete floor and expected the worst, but my body felt remarkable, completely free of pain. I was at peace. I realized I was still alive and felt a deep sense that all of my maladies would heal. Although the mosquitos were gone, my skin was covered with little red tattoos, like a bad case of measles. For days after, they were reminders of the whole surreal experience and of the unforeseen forms that grace takes when it lifts us from despair.

~

A healing crisis had passed, and it now seemed possible that I could move on from the chaos and disorientation of Shandor's departure. Soon, new twists on my journey—the first of these occurring on that same trip to India—would afford me glimpses of my new yoga path: one that expanded the definition of a *body* engaged in yoga *asana* beyond the physical anatomy and into subtle realms.

But the subtle world had spoken to me before, though I didn't recognize it for what it was at the time. For that first discovery, let me take you back to the beginning . . .

And what might seem to be a series
of unfortunate events may, in fact,
be the first steps of a journey.

**Lemony Snicket**

2

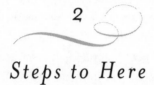

*Steps to Here*

How are we drawn to yoga, and what is it about yoga that sticks? The unique circumstances that lead any of us to our first yoga class are some of life's many mysteries. Is it destiny or perhaps an unfortunate event such as illness or injury that brings yoga to our doorstep? In my case, it was a little of both.

I was born in the 1950s, the middle child in a conservative, first-generation immigrant family living a middle-class life in a small agricultural town in California's Central Valley. On both sides of the family, my grandparents had fled war, forgoing the only life and traditions that generations of their ancestors had ever known. The lessons of those wrenching experiences were passed down to my parents. Planning for many possibilities—especially bad ones—was deeply implanted as a necessity of life, and my brothers and I were raised to set goals and make plans. My father talked constantly about the strategies he used to get through life:

- "Always have a plan . . . or two."

- "Prepare for the worst but expect the best."

- "Never be complacent."

- "Always be moving forward and never quit."

- "Obstacles are opportunities."

By the time I graduated from high school in 1974, I couldn't wait to leave home, driven not by those incessant messages or by the teenage angst most of my friends felt while being trapped in what amounted to a real-life movie set of *American Graffiti,* but by a personal curiosity and deep desire to experience life on my own, beyond the comfortable shelter of family and friends.

During my senior year, I applied and was accepted to a university on the coast (far enough from home to suit me), where I would study architecture, absorbing the foundational principles of the field and exploring their edges. Some of those principles, I would later learn, also apply to yoga.

And it was there at the university that I had my first taste of the yoga path.

## PEEKING THROUGH A DOOR

I woke up late for class as usual, having stayed up until 4:00 a.m. to finish a project that was due later that morning. True to my father's advice, I was always pushing forward, hard. I had only slept three hours in that past forty-eight, and my whole body ached, especially my neck. As I passed through the rec center on my way to class, I noticed the door to a group fitness room was propped open just enough to peek inside. To this day, I don't know why I had the impulse to stop, turn, and look in. But when I did, what I saw made no sense to me. With no context from previous life experience to draw from, it was as though I'd just landed in another world and was witnessing some strange ritual performed by an alien species of being. Even stranger, I found myself pushing open the door and walking in, entering a room full of girls exercising.

"Can I help you?" the teacher asked, her voice inviting.

"What is this?" I asked.

"It's a yoga class."

"What's that?"

"If you'd like to find out, you're welcome to join."

Oh, no—that was not what I was expecting to hear. Put on the spot, I was suddenly embarrassed, until I noticed that most of the faces focused on me held warm looks of encouragement and welcome.

"Sure," I decided. "When's the next class?"

A week later, I was back, looking silly, no doubt, in tennis shoes, white athletic socks, and basketball shorts, shirtless, with my long '70s hair pulled back with a sweatband for "coolness," like I was ready for a workout in the weight room next door.

The class started with all of us on the floor sitting still, cross-legged. The teacher began to chant Sanskrit, and everyone except me tried to follow—some more successfully than others. Luckily the chanting didn't last long, and soon the instructor had us stand up for a sequence of poses she called "Salutations to the Sun." I thought, *I can do this—I really like the sun!*

My first set of the sequence was humbling. It was a fully self-conscious process, but not in the yogic sense—more in the egotistical sense: *Am I doing it "right"? How come I can't touch my toes like they do? Did she say left foot or right foot? Is that my left foot? What is a perineum? Is that sweat on my mat, or am I drooling? Holy crap, this is harder than I thought! How many more of these are we going to do?*

After three rounds of salutations, I was dripping in sweat and breathing like I'd scaled a Himalayan peak without oxygen. I felt like I was going to pass out. But then the pace of the class slowed down. We did a short series of floor poses—gentle twists and seated forward bends—which I could only access using straps for clasping my feet and a bolster under my butt to elevate my hips. Each pose inched me closer to the sheer agony of fully stretching my chronically tight hamstrings. The pain was intense; I imagined this must be what childbirth felt like. Fortunately, the instructor came over and adjusted my pose; with her guidance, the pain dialed back a notch. I gained a little confidence that the pain response in my legs could be eased with the help of calm touch.

When we finished the last set of poses, we were asked to lie down on our backs and close our eyes. The teacher led us though a relaxation exercise, where we moved our attention to various parts of our bodies, alternately squeezing and releasing different muscle groups from head to toe. After the last release, she asked us to bring our awareness to the breath and just follow the rise and fall of the lungs. Where I went after that I have no idea. The next thing I consciously knew was a gentle touch on my shoulder to wake me up. The class was over, and half the people had already left.

"How was that?" the instructor asked.

I could only smile. The miserable ache in my neck that I had come in with from the previous week, studying like a maniac for two days straight with little sleep, was gone. In fact, all my usual aches and pains were gone. I was hooked!

## TWISTS AND TURNS

My journey from that first class to Shandor was circuitous and filled with improbable—sometimes outright ridiculous—coincidences. It was as though a path were somehow being cleared between us, although it still held its own obstacles in store.

After graduating with my architecture degree in 1980, I spent the summer helping a friend build his house on Puget Sound in Washington. Over breakfast one morning, paging through the *Seattle Times*, I spotted a microscopic ad for a yearlong position on the East Coast, working full time in the National Park Service, for anyone with a degree in architecture, no experience required. It was as if the writer of the ad had been looking at my life and résumé when creating it: Architecture degree? Check. No experience? Check. Able to relocate quickly? Check. Gets Dad off my back about a "real job"? Checkmate!

Within a month of being hired, I boarded a train heading from Philadelphia to New York and looked for an empty seat in the overly crowded car—even the aisles were stuffed with "suits." Remarkably, I found one and, even more remarkably, a pretty girl with luminous green eyes in the seat next to me. The next two hours flew by, our time together filled with our life stories, and when we parted the train, she placed a scrap of paper in my hand with her phone number scribbled on it. The year went by quickly, and I soon followed her to Santa Fe, a place unknown to me, and found work my second day there in an architectural firm—but with a strange requirement: the job was mine if I joined the local rugby team. That's right, rugby. I knew nothing about the sport, but I must have looked the part. It was a dream job and my first opportunity to design real buildings. On the rugby side of the arrangement, our team, mostly former collegiate athletes, made its unlikely way into a national tournament—and won.

As a result of our success, the team was invited to tour New Zealand. I jumped at the chance to go, as the romance that had taken me to New Mexico had ended sooner than I had expected.

I was packing up my things ahead of the trip and happened upon some old architecture magazines I subscribed to. As I thumbed through one trying to decide whether to keep or toss it, a tiny employment ad caught my eye . . . déjà vu. This job was for an architectural consultant in Auckland, New Zealand. I tore out the page, folded it neatly, and put it in my wallet, hopeful that it would come in handy soon. The first thought of staying in New Zealand for longer than just the tour was born.

In New Zealand, more head-shaking encounters marked my path. In a needle-in-a-haystack moment, map in hand and looking confused while standing on a busy Auckland street corner, I was approached by a man with an obvious American accent, wondering if I needed help finding something. I told him I was looking for a company and pulled the ad from my wallet. The guy not only knew where the company was, but he also knew the owner! He offered to make introductions, and we walked there together, just two blocks away.

I didn't get that job, and I wondered if synchronistic events had steered me wrong for a change. But within minutes of my learning the job had been filled, the American decided to hire me himself.

Another haystack needle appeared when my new boss hosted an end-of-summer party. While there, I met a professor of architecture from the University of Auckland. When I shared that my first job out of architecture school had been in Santa Fe, the gentleman grew excited, describing with great enthusiasm, and in uncanny detail, the design of a church he had recently read about in an article, one he greatly admired despite never having seen it in person. Turns out, it was the first structure I had designed that was built!

With the professor as my sponsor, I began lecturing part time at the university. That job, in turn, led me, four months later, to another teaching position, full time, this one in the city of Wellington, and at long last . . .

. . . into a yoga studio with Shandor Remete.

## "I'M NOT SURE I'VE LEARNED YOGA"

On my first day of work in Wellington, I had lunch at a quaint neighborhood cafe. On its community board was a flier, nearly buried under others like it, for a weekly yoga class that, as luck would have it, was at a small elementary school near my house. Bingo! While I had continued to study the philosophy of yoga in Auckland in old books I found in the university library, classes had been hard to find, and I was eager to find a teacher.

When I arrived for class, the room was full of women (again), but this time I felt at home. My personal practice was producing results, and I felt no timidity being the only "somewhat stiff" guy in the room. After class, the teacher introduced herself and asked where I had learned yoga. My answer was odd: "I'm not sure I've learned yoga yet."

In that moment, I think she recognized something similar in me to her teacher, and she suggested I come to a special workshop she was hosting for him. She handed me a flier to take home. The photo at the top captivated me. It was of a muscular man doing an extreme yoga pose with one leg behind his head. I could see he possessed incredible athletic ability, as well as a self-assured presence and maturity that were alluring.

Then I read the workshop description. Damn, this was going to be one boot camp–like weekend: four 4-hour classes over Saturday and Sunday with a 2-hour lecture and demonstration on Friday night.

Shandor Remete's bio was intimidating; this guy had been a soldier in the Australian army and a member of a special forces unit in Vietnam. He was a black belt in martial arts, had started yoga with his father when he was six, and for the past twenty-five years had learned some very extreme techniques from a yoga master in India—the revered B. K. S. Iyengar. He oozed machismo. Everything about him was virile, and it drew me in. I was the opposite on almost every front. I lacked a strong masculine sense of myself. Having grown up during the early days of the women's liberation movement of the 1960s, I considered myself a pacifist and a peacemaker. I was not a big fan of testosterone.

The Friday night demonstration he gave was like a contortionist freak show—I was almost revulsed. *What am I doing here?* I thought. But then he began to talk, and his lecture was fascinating. He spoke about things I'd never heard of before. He talked about balance between our physical and psychological bodies and their inseparable nature. He talked about life force, or *prana*, a new term for me, and how, with the regular practice of yoga, it would flow through us with ease and strength, allowing us to become masters of our emotions and our afflictions. Surprisingly, he was soft spoken, with a thick Hungarian accent that was both mysterious and hard to understand at times. Yet his presence was magnetic.

The first class Saturday morning started with a thirty-minute seated meditation. Initially, gentle postural guidance for efficient sitting was interspersed with philosophical concepts. Then we sat in absolute silence, listening only to the sound of our breath. We were forbidden from moving—anyone who budged in the slightest was scolded: "Don't fidget." Having never sat absolutely still in my life, I was a constant target for his theatrical wrath, or so it seemed.

Then we stood up, and he moved us in and out of poses nonstop for the next two and a half hours. Although it was strenuous, his vehement tone and the subliminal threat of humiliation if I quit kept an intravenous drip of adrenaline flowing and gave me the stamina to carry on.

For the last thirty minutes, we did a cooldown form of practice of head and shoulder stand variations, followed by seated forward bends, and ending with a supine relaxation pose.

It was in this final pose that I experienced for the first time a clear separation of mind from body. My body was in a corpse-like state; the feeling of relaxation was so deep, I felt like none of my limbs would move even if my mind willed them to. And yet, another part of my mind was aware and conscious of a subtle cerebral process that felt completely at ease with the situation, simultaneously full of life force mentally and devoid of life force physically.

During the break between classes that first day, I was among the few students Shandor invited to join him for lunch, and I was the only new student. Meeting him this way, I saw his personal side, which brought him down to an approachable level. Since I was the only American in class and he had not yet been to the States to teach, he was genuinely interested in hearing about my life and was happy to share a few of his life stories. This would be the beginning of my twenty-year relationship studying with him.

The weekend was life altering, sparking a passion for yoga that felt like it would always be there. And except for a few unexpected sabbaticals, over the next thirty-five years, that passion remained true.

## TEACHINGS OF THE MASTER

During the first few years, my opportunities to study with Shandor were limited to his annual visits to New Zealand. When he was in Wellington, I attended every class, showing up early to set up my mat, front and center, to observe every detail of his demonstrations and clearly hear his every word. My notebooks were filled with pages and pages of scribble, trying to keep up with his voice. After classes, a few of us met for tea to write down what we could remember of the practice sequences, hoping in the end to have a script to help us re-create the correct order and reexperience the incredible feelings that resulted—all this despite him telling us not to be too concerned with taking notes.

"Trust your listening. Have faith in what you hear and see. Do only what you remember and keep practicing regularly. The seeds of my words and the feeling of each pose have been planted in you. Regular practice and consistent study will eventually provide the ground for intelligence to unfold." Initially, this advice was frustrating, memory not being one of my strong suits. But over the next five years, practicing with him once a year, the wisdom in his advice became self-evident.

Early on, I didn't understand that the effects I felt during his classes had less to do with an individual pose or the particular sequence they were a part of and more to do with his skill in directing our attention to the present moment, where we were more receptive to subtle influences, whether watching him or practicing ourselves. This principle is key to the approach you will learn in this book.

## THE ENERGY OF TRANSMISSION

Seeing Shandor move entailed much more than watching. My experience as he moved through his practice, and especially when he did the advanced practices he didn't teach in his workshops, inspired me. And that inspiration seemed to come to me through senses other than sight. I listened to his gentle, undisturbed breathing. I felt his presence moving in and out of poses, and I noticed where in my own body those feelings arose. At times, my mind was confused by demanding poses that he made look effortless, and at other times, when his effort was more obvious, he held a quality of undisturbed equanimity. He was fully present in his moment, with an aura of deep stillness, emotionally and intellectually, no matter what he was doing on his mat. He was in the zone, and I felt its effects on me—like a transmission of presence between us, as if my body were experiencing a virtual practice through his own.

I felt inside my body an invitation to move into the spaces these feelings were naturally creating: feelings of softness, openness, and calm. It took me another decade working on my own to understand how the process worked and then to develop a vocabulary for my own inner process that I could use in teaching.

At the time of these experiences with Shandor, I had never heard of a subtle body entwined with the physical body. But even then, I was waking to the mysteries of it.

## BREAKING THE RULES

Fast-forward to now. Twenty years after my first experience of these subtle levels of being with Shandor, two things happened in quick succession that helped me integrate my subtle body education more personally.

The first took place at the Ayurvedic hospital in the aftermath of my split with Shandor. So, let's return to India for a brief moment, before moving on to the States.

During the last week of my hospital stay, a nurse who had heard I was a yoga teacher offered to show me the hospital's yoga studio. It was a nondescript room, much like the one I was staying in, with a collection of old black-and-white photos hung high on the walls for the practicing students to see. The model in the pictures was a trim, middle-aged man doing very unusual poses, many of which I had never seen before. I inquired whether I could attend classes for my remaining time there but was told the teacher only taught schoolchildren. I insisted (as a child would) and was finally told to show up the next day to ask the guru for permission.

In the morning, I arrived early and found a room full of young boys waiting patiently for class to begin. They giggled nervously at the sight of a Western man carrying a yoga mat, and when the teacher arrived, there was dead silence. He was much older than the man on the walls and spoke in a language foreign to me. Then one of the boys translated in perfect English that he was welcoming me to class and was honored with my presence. For the next two hours, with not a word spoken that I understood, I did my best to mimic what I saw the children doing.

Over the next six days, those kids were my teacher as they performed unusual sequences of unusual poses effortlessly, without yoga mats, on a very hard marble floor. There was no struggle or hesitation. I felt only infectious joy and clear reverence for the master, who was lighthearted, generous, and kind. As I watched the boys practice, I saw body shapes and movements that were entirely different—even "wrong"—compared to what I had been taught the physical poses of yoga were supposed to look like. All at once, I had an inkling of what would bring me back to yoga.

# CIRQUE

The experience with the boys was soon reinforced after I returned home to California to find a single message on my answering machine, from an old friend in New Mexico. Naturally intuitive, she had felt moved to reconnect after many years. If I felt the same, she asked, could I meet her halfway in Las Vegas for the weekend? Both her timing and tone were perfect, and I accepted. In that glittering city, devoid of anything yogic in those days, I would take the next unplanned step in my subtle body education.

For our first night there, she had purchased tickets for Cirque du Soleil, with seats three rows back from the stage. From that vantage, the dancers' movements and breathing imprinted powerfully on my nervous system. I was in awe of the grace and effortless power their bodies displayed, and the yoga teacher in me analyzed every aspect: the curvaceous ways their spines moved in any direction, the smooth quality of their muscle tissue, the fluidity of their breath, the peaceful expressions on their faces, the soft suppleness of their skin. And something else . . . a mysterious quality of movement that was vaguely familiar, something I had seen before but couldn't put a finger on at first.

During the intermission, it came to me. I was witnessing the same thing the schoolboys at the hospital had displayed in class. Every rule of "correct" body alignment I'd been taught in my twenty years in yoga was being broken; yet both the dancers and the boys created a joyful sense of movement that was not only graceful but also safe. They were breaking the so-called rules without hurting themselves.

As I sat watching the second act with a more critical eye, I felt sensations throughout my body that were viscerally connected to the dancers' bodies. Some sense organ other than my eyes was receiving tele-somatic signals directly from their movements. My mind recognized where those internal sensations were flowing, guided through distinct channels (*nadis*) and concentrating in various locations (*chakras*) of my subtle body (*suksma sarira*).

I could feel my desire to practice yoga again growing. My excitement to roll out my mat was back.

## A BEGINNER AGAIN

Back home and returning to practice, I began revisiting old techniques I had already learned as if seeing them for the first time. Techniques I had taken for granted, usually borrowed from others, became foreign to my new understanding, like old souvenirs from a forgotten place. My return to yoga started by acknowledging all the experiences of my previous practice—successful or not, right or wrong, breakthroughs or breakdowns—as useful for the next steps of my yoga journey. How could they not be? What evolved from this realization was a different way to approach physical (*hatha*) yoga. I would come to each practice as a beginner again, with a sense of deep curiosity and presence to the subtle sensations that showed up through movement, breath, and stillness, surrendering to the experience of things as they appeared. Seeing for myself, with as much joy and lightheartedness as possible, became fundamental to my practice, free of any attachment to, or bias of, my teachers.

I also set out to discover what was no longer serving my next steps forward and to eliminate what was nonessential to this new way of practicing. This was mostly a trial-and-error process. Starting on my mat, I would feel an intuitive urge to drop a particular movement or pose; I would then work without it for a while and patiently wait for intuition to offer an alternative that would let me move beyond what I had known. When uncertainty arose or nothing clear appeared intuitively, I accepted not knowing in that moment and continued practicing. Frequently, at these mysterious pauses in moving forward, seemingly random books or articles appeared, often having nothing explicitly to do with yoga, offering timely contributions to support going further. These synchronistic events were one of the many forms of grace.

Within a few months of consistently practicing in this way, I came to trust the process and understand how to apply the insights that resulted. I learned to recognize patterns—which first appeared while practicing and later echoed in other aspects of my life—that supported this new way of moving forward. The best times to identify these patterns were during periods of mental calm and physical stillness—states that allowed me to see things from a perspective that was detached from ordinary thinking. In those moments, I had glimpses that what I had thought was "me" was not who I really was.

To discard those things that did not serve my new, expanded perception, I developed two questions to test whether what I was doing served a deeper purpose: First, is the experience I'm having—whether through reading, watching, listening, or practicing—helping me be more genuinely present with myself and with others in my life? And second, is what I am seeing or hearing in this experience true?

I also developed a few principles of practice, which I will share with you in part 5 of this book, to help maintain presence, whether in movement or stillness, and to improve my ability to be with any discomfort that arose in either—to touch, or acknowledge, that sensation as softly as possible. Teaching yoga students to move or be this way has refined my understanding of how this level of presence can work in any situation, at any moment. It can also help us drop the expectations that come from—and are intrinsically part of—following.

In the pursuit of knowledge, every day something is added. In the practice of the Tao [intelligence], every day something is dropped.

**Lao Tzu**

Being cut loose from the apprenticeship that had defined yoga practice for me for so many years had freed me to find my own way and to discover that no matter how we find yoga—or how it improbably finds us—we all come to yoga as we are, accompanied by the best teacher we could ever have: the teacher within. With this book, I aim to give you the tools you need to hear that inner teacher and the encouragement to let it guide you.

Miracles . . . rest not so much upon faces or voices
or healing power coming suddenly new to us
from afar off, but upon perceptions being made
finer, so that for the moment our eyes can see and
our ears can hear what is there about us always.

**Willa Cather**

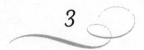

# 3

# *Embracing the Unexpected*

In this chapter, I want to take you deeper into the ways the subtle body can be awakened through the practice of yoga. As you will soon see, I learned the principles I introduce here the hard way, but fortunately, you won't have to. As you absorb them, I encourage you to begin experimenting with them intuitively in your own practice. In part 5, I will give you detailed instruction in how to incorporate these concepts into some common yoga poses.

In 1993, after living out of the country for more than ten years, the time had arrived for me to return to the United States. Yoga's popularity was flourishing across the country, with classes now easily found in most major cities. With a growing student base, the American yoga industry was ramping up: there were branded studios, products, clothing, teacher training schools, and even a dedicated magazine full of celebrity teachers and mainstream endorsements. While in India, yoga remained mostly discreet and hidden from popular culture, in America, the commercial genie was out of the bottle.

I was back in California, which was fast becoming a mecca for American yoga. I had moved to San Luis Obispo, where I'd attended university and which, surprisingly, had no yoga studio. Although teaching wasn't on my radar, within a few months of my return, a handful of friends were asking me to teach. One of them had connections at a senior center two blocks from my house, so I started teaching on the only evening of the week without a bingo class.

My early students helped spread fliers around town; in a very short time, word was out, and the class was full. As forgettable as those early classes were, they were deeply appreciated by those who came, curious about yoga and seeking instruction from a teacher who'd actually studied in India.

Soon we were outgrowing the senior center, and I found a new, larger space (completely derelict and vacant for two decades) downtown. After "a little" renovating, it was perfect for a yoga studio, and in February 1994, we opened. Through word of mouth, free ads in the local paper, and fliers posted everywhere, the first yoga studio in town was a hit. Our new yoga community not only supported our vision but also grew it in ways I never could have imagined.

## DANCING WITH A BEAR

As the holidays approached at the end of our first year, our plan was to close the studio until the New Year. As a compromise to our dedicated students, we offered a special holiday class one evening that I co-taught with another instructor. Each of us would take turns teaching while the other assisted, moving about the room to adjust and support beginning students' poses as needed.

The other teacher went first, and after an initial series of very simple poses, I was surprised when she had students attempt a wall-supported handstand. As I watched many beginners' first attempts to kick their legs up the wall, I suddenly had frightening visions of students falling like dominoes. Almost immediately, on the opposite side of the room, I noticed a large bear of a man, upside down, with his legs awkwardly placed up the wall. His arms were strong, but they were bent slightly and shaking uncontrollably. As he appeared on the verge of collapse, I sprinted across the room without a thought, praying that I would reach him before his head was rudely introduced to the floor.

The rest unfolded in slow motion. His arms buckled as I lurched forward and reached to catch his hips and break his fall. We both went down together, and I heard a sound I never expected that night, like a thick bone breaking or dislocating. I was sure the student's neck or back had broken or his skull had cracked, and I jumped to my feet in shock.

"Are you okay?"

He was conscious—and clearly embarrassed. Red-faced, he answered, "I'm fine." A torrent of relief flushed through me, and I thought how lucky the student and our new studio had been in that moment, dodging a "breakneck" bullet.

But the night was still young, and the adrenaline coursing in my bloodstream was starting to wane.

Once the class resumed, I moved next to a student struggling with balance in a beginner-appropriate standing pose and applied a simple adjustment, one I'd done a thousand times without incident. As I leaned in to adjust, pain shot up my spine like a bolt of lightning hurled from the ground, and my back locked up completely. Frozen in a semi-hunched-forward position, I couldn't move—or breathe. The slightest movement, even a normal breath, brought agony. I now knew that the bone-breaking sound I had heard had come from me.

I wondered what to do next. Nearby was a knee-high stage that offered me a possible place to rest. Shuffling backward with baby steps and even smaller breaths—and too self-conscious to ask for help—I managed to reach the edge of the stage and awkwardly (that would be an understatement), painfully (another understatement) lowered myself onto it. I signaled to the other instructor that I was unable to teach, so she finished for me.

After class, a fellow teacher drove me home and helped me into my house. Even assisted, walking to my upstairs bedroom was impossible, so the downstairs family room became my living space.

I had thought I'd sleep on the couch, but no matter the position, my lower back was having none of it. Intuitively, I began testing a variety of sleeping positions on the floor using various yoga props I had lying around the house. Despite taking multiple over-the-counter painkillers, the only position I found remotely bearable was prone, kneeling, with my chest and belly firmly supported on a high stack of stiff sofa cushions and my head turned to one side, resting on a small pillow. This put my legs in a slight state of traction from my pelvis, which took some of the pressure off my lower back. I could maintain this position—basically, an elevated Child's Pose—for hours at a time. This was my existence for the next twelve days, floor-ridden.

The first night, I didn't sleep a lot, not so much because of the pain but because my mind was in overdrive, worried about the long-term effects of this injury and how it would impact my ability to practice and teach yoga.

In the morning, I called an orthopedic surgeon. He ordered a series of MRIs, and the results he shared in his office days later were not good. Pointing to a large, conveniently placed poster on his treatment room wall, the surgeon showed me how a ruptured disc in the lumbar area of my spine was putting pressure on the sciatic nerve and how fluid leaking through the tear in the disc cartilage was also increasing pressure inside the spinal canal, likely contributing to nerve inflammation and more pain.

After breaking all that news, what he said next—in a less-than-comforting way, I'd add—was unbearable: "In cases like this, surgery is really the only course of action to remove the bulging disc tissue that's pressing against the spinal cord. Without surgery, re-injury and a lifetime of back problems are highly likely."

All the helpful people in my life strongly encouraged me to listen to the doctors and have the surgery—all, that is, except one. I called Shandor to get his take on what I should do. I explained precisely what had happened, including the position I had been in as I fully embraced the bottom half of my upside-down, 230-pound dance partner. With my teacher's calm assurance of what to do next, I came away from the call with a sliver of hope.

What Shandor said made sense. Since the injury occurred in a forward bending position, the posterior side of the disc had popped backward, oozing out like the bubble that forms when a child squeezes a slime ball. He felt confident that with *gentle* movement in the other direction, the pressure on the disc would reverse, and the "slime" would eventually gravitate back in—or at least wouldn't leak further. With time, the tear would heal, and fluid within the disc would regenerate.

"How much time?" I asked.

His reply was depressing: "Twelve to eighteen months. But for now, just rest, drink lots of water, and do heaps of *pranayama* [the breathing practices I had learned from him] until you can fully stand."

## RECOVERY . . . AND DISCOVERY: SEEDS OF GRAVITY AND GRACE

My days propped on the stack of cushions were filled with books about spine rehabilitation, conscious breathing exercises, and not much else. After two weeks spent floor-bound, crawling everywhere I had to go downstairs, I was finally able to sit upright for brief periods, and I could finally go upstairs to sleep in a bed.

I began a simple routine of yoga poses during my waking hours—restorative poses only, which would take pressure off my lower back. I drew on a pose involving a folding chair I'd learned while studying in India at the Iyengar Institute. I would lay supine, with my legs bent and supported on the seat of a chair with a folded hand towel and with a rolled-up washcloth to support my lumbar and cervical vertebrae, respectively. This setup completely pacified all of the paraspinal nerves and muscles of my back. I would stay in this position for twenty minutes or more, at least three to four times a day.

While resting in the pose, focusing on slow, conscious breathing, I began to notice two things: first, there was a difference in the levels of pain I felt when inhaling and exhaling; and second, any sensation I was feeling seemed to follow where I placed my attention. I had no idea at the time that I was learning some of the foundational applications of gravity and grace I would later teach.

> The *hsin* (mind)
> mobilizes the *ch'i* (breath).
>
> Make the *ch'i* sink calmly;
> then it gathers
> and permeates the bones.
>
> The *ch'i* mobilizes the body.
>
> Make it flow smoothly,
> then it easily follows
> the direction of the *hsin*.
>
> Wu Yu-hsiang

On the inhale, I felt the subtle expansion of my lungs creating a very slight spike of pain in the lower back and down my left leg, as the diaphragm contracted and pressed down against my abdominal organs. When my breath was deep, the pain was more intense; when it was shallow, the pain was much less. On the exhale, whether my breath was deep or shallow, there was a noticeable reduction in pain as my diaphragm released its muscular grip on my ribs and lower back, and I felt the gentle softening of my belly as the intercavity pressure of the abdomen dropped. Over days, I came to realize that if I spent less time inhaling and more time exhaling, the amount of time I was in pain would lessen. This, I thought, might give my parasympathetic nervous system more time to go to work on releasing the residue of subconscious contraction still present from the initial trauma of my injury, which was keeping up a chronic level of stimulus in my sympathetic nervous system.

The more time I spent breathing like this, not only did I feel stronger, but I also felt as if I was consciously participating in my body's self-healing. Using only my breath to activate subtle physical sensations beyond the boundaries of my lungs, I could focus my attention and initiate subtle movement in the injured part of my spine. Over many weeks of observing this process, I became aware that placing my attention into my pain and connecting the subtle sensations of breath to where my attention was placed lessened my discomfort and helped support my body's capacity to heal on its own.

Each day brought new insights. I realized that breathing slowly was more effective than breathing deeply, especially on the inhale. The longer I took to reach a comfortable lung capacity without overexpanding my rib cage, the more satisfying and effortless my exhales were in reducing pain. This allowed me to gradually overcome the obvious limitations of breathing shallowly to deal with the immediate problem of severe pain—after all, that strategy had not taken into account the body's need for adequate oxygen when inhaling and the mental anxiety produced by shortness of breath.

Breathing slowly allowed me to transcend breathing shallowly. I visualized my breath as if I were inhaling one molecule of oxygen at a time. As long as I was aware of air coming in, the mental component of breathing was satisfied that my respiration needs were being met (albeit very slowly); this allowed me to continue inhaling gently until my lungs were comfortably full and the physical component of my breath was satisfied. Having an ease-full lung to exhale with allowed the duration of my outgoing breath to feel endless.

I gradually increased the amount of time I engaged this practice, which eventually increased my pain-free time dramatically. How this worked, exactly, was a mystery then, but I had no doubt that conscious breathing was playing a big role.

As I got better at inhaling with minimal pain, I noticed pleasurable sensations throughout my body with every exhale, as my nervous system fully relaxed. It started in the belly. As my diaphragm released on the exhale, I felt an inner spaciousness opening in the abdomen. Even though my abdominal wall was physically receding on the exhale, the subtle sensations of my breath were creating an abounding feeling of "inner space" in my gut and a deep sense of softness in the connective tissue supporting my body's internal organs and bones. I also noticed that as the diaphragm released, the weight of my abdominal organs dropped, which produced a subtle vacuum and an emptiness like that of "outer space" on a clear, star-lit night,which I could sense in the gut.

As I began to explore being upright again, the sensation of my abdominal organs sinking also caused a feeling of heaviness in my pelvic floor that produced a physical and psychological sense of grounding and comfort. What I didn't fully understand then, I would discover many years later from my medical research on the effects of healthy vagal nerve tone—that is, slow (not deep) breathing affects the role that the vagus nerve plays in stimulating the parasympathetic nervous system and, ultimately, the immune system's ability to reduce inflammation, which is one of the primary sources of pain and disease in the body.

~

And now the story changes. After only four weeks—nowhere close to my worst fears—I was able to move with a large degree of normalcy. I went back to work and began teaching again.

Much more than my breathing had changed during that time. I had also gained the capacity to be present with the simplest things. Authentic humility had asserted itself into my daily routine and in so many aspects of my life where previously there had been very little or none. I became more sensitive to how I positioned myself when working at a drafting table, sitting in front of a computer, or even lounging on the couch watching TV. In yoga, I still avoided practicing forward bends or twists of any kind (standing, sitting, or reclining), though I now possessed a whole new respect for how vulnerable the lower back could be. This awareness profoundly influenced how I taught students with limited mobility, especially of the legs, hips, or back.

Meanwhile, I was seriously questioning the ways I had moved in the past, especially during yoga in standing forward bends: "Chest up, arms out, chin forward, folding at the hips, 'swan dive' forward, flat back." How many times had I heard that in class as a way to keep the spine safe, let alone repeated it when teaching myself? It was time to question all the rules.

## GRAVITY AND GRACE INSIGHTS DEEPEN

After half a year, the passive quality of my practice naturally began to change. The ease I felt with gentle, gravity-assisted back bending inspired the introduction of more dynamic backbends, although with a profound respect for what I had learned from conscious breathing and stillness. Unless I could maintain the subtle space I felt while exhaling, I would not engage my poses any further. And since inhaling tended to produce pain, another realization appeared: the inhalation cycle would now be the *ebb cycle* of my poses—a momentary pause in the process of moving deeper with my body and my mind—and the *flow cycle* of my poses would be on the exhalation, when the inner spaciousness to move appeared naturally.

It went even further. As I allowed myself to feel the subtle expansion of inhaling, a somatic sense of buoyancy created a lift physically, as if I were coming out, quite literally, of whatever pose I was in. This made so much sense to me because *hatha* yoga is a discipline of effort and challenge interwoven with non-effort and ease. Coming out of my poses slightly with the passive influence provided by each inhale created a profound realization for a chronic doer like me. The buoyancy it created gave me a sense of lightness physically and mentally, a sense of levity; it reset my nervous system with a parasympathetic current of relaxation and presence.

With my back feeling stronger, curiosity awakened a desire to do forward bends again; it was time to test what my back injury had taught me so far. I started with the simplest forward bend I knew: lying flat on my back, with the lumbar and cervical curves of my spine supported, one leg lifted and supported by a yoga strap looped around my foot and held in my hands. In this position, the pain in my mildly stretching hamstring was manageable. But this time, the goal was not to stretch; it was to see if the technique I used to mitigate pain in my back could be used for the discomfort I was feeling in my hamstring.

From the very first breath, I was awed by what happened. Since I was hypersensitive to the possibility of re-injuring my back, keeping my mind present with the sensation of my breath as it moved down along the spine occurred naturally. In this pose, if my inhale and the subsequent subtle movement it created caused any hint of pain in my spine where the herniated disc was weakened, it became an inviolable indication that my pose was too extreme and served as a signal to back off the stretch a little.

Then, unexpectedly, I started making the acquaintance of a fundamental system of the subtle body.

## *CHAKRAS* GET REAL

As I followed the sensations of my breath slowly moving through the nasal passages and down through my back, I became aware of subconscious tension that hovered around other, less familiar landmarks near my spine: the back of my throat/root of my tongue (cervical); the back of my heart (thoracic); the diaphragm and back of my abdomen (upper and middle lumbar); the bladder and back of my rectum (sacrum); and finally, into the root of the genitals and pelvic floor (coccyx). I realized that the proximity of these areas of subliminal gripping happened to be areas of great importance to both ancient and modern-day yogis—the so-called vortexes of subtle body energy known as *chakras*.

Until then, I had been unaware a relationship existed between these two concepts within our subtle bodies—the places of subconscious gripping resulting from the various stressors or traumas (psychological and physical) in life and the powerful seats of various subtle energies that were to be channeled, toned, and used for spiritual development in *hatha* yoga.

Much later, through more research, I was surprised to learn that the body's endocrine system has its own set of glandular plexuses located in close proximity to the nerve and *chakra* network nodes in the body. The endocrine glandular system is instrumental in regulating mood, growth and development, tissue function, and metabolism by secreting hormones and other biochemical agents that support healthy cellular functioning and suppleness throughout the body, including our organs, muscles, and the web of connective tissue that interlinks almost everything inside the outer layer of our skin.

Meanwhile, back at my forays of easing into forward bends, astonishing discoveries appeared to me. With each exhale, as I anticipated the release I had experienced when recuperating my lower back, I intuitively sensed that if I could first release subconscious holding around blocked or stiff areas of my back, the overall effect on my nervous system—in particular, the parasympathetic—might produce a similar effect on my endocrine system; combined, they might release whatever subconscious holding chronically resided in the connective tissue that encased and interwove the muscles of my lower trunk and hamstrings.

You will learn much more about the principles behind these discoveries further along in this book.

# PART 2

## *The Energies of Gravity and Grace*

In part 1, I walked you through key experiences that led me to the approach to yoga that honors each practitioner's unique body and mind, in each present moment, while activating awareness of subtle body energies. You now know how it happened that a determined—okay, maybe even obsessive—devotee of a rigorous, exacting style of yoga came to teach a fluid, intuitive form of practice that is never the same two days in a row. I have also acquainted you with some of the key elements of this approach—the way they might show up in real life. Now let's take a deeper dive into the principles of gravity and grace and explore how they might apply to your yoga practice and your life.

When the outward form shows man's right
relationship with himself, he appears
both held and released, self-contained yet
animated by a living dynamism, tensed and
relaxed in a right alternation and balance.

**Karlfried Graf Dürckheim**

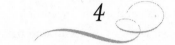

# Effort and Non-Effort

## FATHER CHARLIE

For many years at our yoga studio, I hosted a visiting spiritual teacher named Charles L. Moore. His life story was as remarkable as his talks. A former district attorney of Santa Cruz County in California, he had left the practice of law and turned his full attention to religious studies, becoming a Roman Catholic priest. With a passion for linguistics, Father Charlie studied Latin and Greek and explored sixteen other languages, including Sanskrit, Sumerian, Chinese, Japanese, Hawaiian, and several Native American languages such as Chumash, Sioux, Blackfoot, and Hopi. He spun elaborate tales of ancient historical events, occasionally speaking as a character in the story he was telling, using the native tongue that he had learned, and then translating into English to make his points more powerful. On special nights, he told stories about moments in our collective human history before civilization—sometimes they were those of legend, and other times they were inspired by his frequent dreams or by his knowledge of archaeological research based on his travels to ancient sites around the world.

Although Father Charlie was not a practicing yogi, he often spoke about the relationship between gravity and grace: how each of these universal forces could be experienced personally in our day-to-day lives. He would start with the gift of gravity, telling us that the creator of our universe had given us gravity for two reasons.

## Grounding, Physically

The first reason for this gift of gravity was to keep us grounded physically, literally keeping us connected to the big ball of dirt, rock, and water we inhabit as it spins and orbits around our sun star, while our solar system of planets and moons orbits around the Milky Way galaxy, and as our galactic system of stars rotates around the center of the universe. The miracle of gravity—revealed by Isaac Newton's apple and the attraction of objects—is its ability to keep our feet on planet Earth while hurtling through space at a staggering speed of 850 kilometers per second (2,000,000 miles per hour).

## Grounding, Psychologically

Father Charlie especially enjoyed describing this second aspect of gravity, which is so essential for the health of our human being. Feeling grounded psychologically allows us to reconnect with our feelings of "home" on this planet. He explored how this natural experience of gravity effortlessly produces its opposite—lightness of heart—in a very similar way to another of Newton's discoveries—the third of three universal laws of motion, which states that for every physical action, there is an equal and opposite reaction.

Father Charlie described the gift of grace as the attraction between spiritual bodies. It is essentially the same as gravity but operating on a different plane—gravity on the physical and grace on the nonphysical. He referenced the science of quantum physics, with its understanding of our reality in other dimensions, and declared, "Gravity operates in 'space-time' and grace operates beyond it."[2] In other words, grace comes from outside the three-dimensional world we know, and gravity operates within. He also pointed out common aspects shared by each force: both are "hidden" or "invisible."

Gravity was unknown to science until its discovery in 1687; today, though still an invisible force, it is well understood and accepted as fact. Grace is still unknown to science, although Father Charlie would say that modern quantum physics is knocking vigorously at the door of discovering that "spirit" is the same energy of attraction that exists between particles at the subatomic level. He hoped that one day soon this would be as well understood and accepted as fact as gravity is today.

By 2003, the concepts of gravity and grace that had been infused in me began to blend with the insights I was uncovering in my yoga practice. I saw how powerful these terms were for conveying subtle body forces during the practice of yoga in a non-esoteric language students could grasp. I was curious to see the effects this type of teaching might produce over time in students at any stage of practice.

## ENTER: LEVITY

Gravity is the root of lightness; stillness,
the ruler of movement.

Lao Tzu

Over many years, I have used the simple terms *gravity* and *grace* to describe two complementary forces of attraction—one physical and one nonphysical—that are useful for safe and efficient movement during the practice of yoga. Both help support us and assist with the release of unwanted, often subconscious, patterns of contraction in our bodies: physical, mental, and emotional. The beauty of applying these two elements in yoga *asana* is their ability to create lightness in the body and mind. To communicate this idea of lightness more efficiently, I searched for a word or term that would effectively and simply capture this feeling of lightness, and through a process that I can only describe as grace, I came back to the word *levity*, which Father Charlie had introduced me to years earlier.

The standard definitions of the word *levity* are lightness in weight; lightness of mind, character, or behavior; or lack of appropriate seriousness or earnestness. These meanings so perfectly capture the dual sense of levity we can experience when practicing *hatha* yoga. When I was in my twenties and thirties, I didn't understand the implications a practice like this would have as I aged. But now that I'm much older, I see the effectiveness of employing a movement practice that reduces unnecessary muscular effort and of holding my attention in any activity with a lighthearted state of mind, relying on my own intuitive sense to respond to the input I receive through the body sensations that my movement creates in real time. Thus I cultivate intelligence and grow from the present-moment experience of my actions, guided in a very personal and sustainable way with a sense of humor and ease. As Glenn Geffcken writes, "Lightness of heart, humor, and even downright silliness can serve as the elixir to resistance."[3]

Since I know that each body is different and we all have a very personal understanding of our lives beyond their physical aspects, what evolved was this new way of using gravity and grace:

- Using gravity as a primary catalyst for movement

- Using grace as a catalyst for inspiration and for strengthening the intuitive parts of our minds

*Gravity*, simply defined, is the attraction of two physical bodies. When practicing yoga, think of yourself as the small body in a permanent state of attraction to the big body, which is the Earth below. Understanding this and experiencing it fully can totally shift the relationship you have with the effort you expend in *asana*. As with all physical things in our universe, when you allow yourself to feel the effects of gravity fully through surrender, it can produce a physical experience of gravity's opposite: levity. The key to experiencing physical lightness when practicing yoga lies in understanding how to respond intuitively when you feel the effects of release of effort.

## GRACE IS ATTRACTION, TOO

Like gravity, the experience of grace also possesses the power to shift how you effort mentally in practice. Think of *grace* simply as an attraction between two bodies that occurs at a level deeper than the physical body—in the subtle body. Consider the elegance of movement you observe in professional dancers or athletes, where effort appears so effortless that it touches something within you, causing an attraction, or chemistry, to occur on an energetic, emotional, or spiritual level.

In a yoga context, the next time you observe an experienced practitioner demonstrating a pose, pay close attention to the feeling center of your heart or any other bodily sensation that arises. Notice any feelings of inspiration, curiosity, or wonder. Make a mental note of what you feel; then, the next time you attempt that pose, focus less on technique or the verbal instruction of a teacher and more on your own experience of the shape you are creating within yourself. See if you can touch your original feelings. Be less concerned with doing the pose "right" and more alert to releasing the unnecessary effort that inhibits your ability to fully *feel* your presence in the pose. When surrender is present and grace is experienced within, consider that what your subtle body is being drawn toward is not so much what you originally experienced watching but more a collective spirit or universal intelligence. We all possess this spirit, which supports us when surrender is present—when self becomes no-self.

The experience of levity while practicing opens you to these types of experiences, where surrender is present within effort, in both the physical and nonphysical properties of gravity and grace. This is a very different way of working compared to common instructions found in styles of yoga that employ strong muscular force and a linear checklist of techniques to create form and movement. The paradox that becomes evident through practicing with the elements of gravity and grace is this: when you release excessive muscular effort, your muscles actually become stronger and suppler.

## SUBTLETIES OF EFFORT AND NON-EFFORT

Fundamental to the practice of yoga that emphasizes the elements of gravity and grace is the interplay between effort and non-effort, a polarity that is reflected in the term *hatha*. This Sanskrit word has many meanings. As with many concepts in yoga, the various translations of numerous scholars are inconsistent and often open to interpretation. In its simplest definition, the word can be broken into two root words: *ha*, meaning "sun," and *tha*, meaning "moon." Many would agree that together, these root words imply a combination or joining of the masculine and feminine principles found in each of us, which commonly symbolizes a union of effort with non-effort, active with passive, and forcefulness with receptivity. Combined with the word *yoga*, we arrive at a definition where, through the practice of *hatha* yoga, we understand and experience simultaneous effort and non-effort through a joining of mind (attention) and movement (action), both actively and passively.

Using awareness of our subtle body, we create a conscious process of joining these concepts in the practice of *asana* by minimizing unnecessary physical effort as a means to increase our life force—one of the main benefits of yoga. It is also a means to identify and activate the subtle forces that operate at a level of awareness deeper than the gross physical body, to create a more efficient way to move. Two of these forces that are most available for practice, especially for beginners, are the subtle energies of gravity and grace. During practice, both are used as objects for our attention and as catalysts for movement, both physically and psychologically.

Another way to look at it is to think of muscles responding to the release of subtle energies, which in turn produces movement created by intuitive invitation, as opposed to muscle-initiated movement created by mental imposition or elaborate practice technique. This view requires a shift in how to effort in practice, with a deeper awareness of these subtle forces in the moment of surrender to keep the body's physical structure from collapsing. Both excessive muscular effort and collapse of the body's anatomical structure can choke or limit the flow of sensation through the subtle channels (*nadis*).

This is where the subtlety of the breath is useful to maintain awareness in the present moment. The breath is an extremely useful tool to show where your mind is or is not during the practice of yoga. When muscular effort is excessive, distortion in breathing is usually the first side effect. Maintaining a smooth, soft, slow rhythm to your breath is a useful reminder not to overwork the muscles.

In all *asana*—standing poses, backbends, forward bends, arm balances, twists, and inversions—the aim is to release unnecessary muscular effort. Surprisingly, letting go of effort requires more finesse than you might expect. In most Western cultures, we've been trained from very early on to rely on muscular effort to create movement and posture. However, if we look at Eastern disciplines such as martial arts or dance, movement is not rooted in muscular force. Instead, movement is rooted in balance (gravity) and in using the elemental forces of nature—earth, water, fire, air, and space/ether. When we understand and experience this, our musculature responds to the movement, instead of the movement responding to the musculature, thus reducing the leakage of muscular energy wasted on excessive effort and the subsequent deterioration of life force.

## GRACE, PRESENCE, AND THE BREATH

As we learn the basics of gravity, grace, and levity, we begin to drop any unnecessary elaboration of movement or breathing. On the physical level, anatomical alignment becomes more intuitive as we consistently return our attention to the spatial experience of our bodies in the gravitational field; this produces an inner response that is expressed in the external form of our bodies. On the nonphysical or subtle body levels, maintaining a present-moment experience of slow, conscious breathing helps keep the mind quiet and helps stimulate the parasympathetic nervous system, producing a calming effect that releases the subconscious muscular contraction in our bodies, which is often produced by a sympathetic nervous system response to the anxiety or stress of doing a pose "right."

Grace requires presence, and it is found within presence itself. When your breath becomes distorted, notice how you become disconnected slightly from the present moment and how your mind drifts, usually into a past or future scenario, like *This can't be good for my body, I can't do this*, or *I'm afraid of getting injured*. Awareness of breathing is one of the most common techniques for keeping the mind in the present moment—the place many spiritual traditions recommend as most optimal for our attention. Being aware of sensation in the body can also generate present-moment experience, as long as there is no story attached to it—that is, when we look at the sensation we're experiencing purely for what it is: a neural-cellular language communicating where imbalance exists in our body. If we can release the story and get beyond the judgment (good or bad) of what happens, sensation is there as our teacher—in a way, it is a gift, speaking to us through the language it uses to invite us into a deeper relationship with a part of ourselves that is out of balance.

And that's all it is. Can you touch that part of yourself even more softly and see what its true nature is? And can you see if it changes? If so, you are working with *hatha*—effort and non-effort, gravity and grace—in the present moment.

If it weren't for the rocks in its bed,
the river would have no song.

**Carl Perkins**

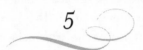

5

# The Hidden Gift of Obstacles

## CONFRONTING YOUR EDGES

We often find metaphors for life in our yoga practice, and those of us who come to yoga stiff or weak are only too familiar with confronting our edges. In most urban, contemporary societies, we are frequently exposed to confrontation: in our communities, our relationships, our jobs—the list goes on. Our success in dealing with confrontation and the stress it generates depends on our ability to recognize and adjust to what presents itself in those situations. It is often easy to avoid dealing with confrontation until it reaches a certain level of intensity and we are forced to address what stands in our way.

When our tools for dealing with confrontation are overwhelmed and when what we perceive as our very nature becomes threatened, our life systems—mental, emotional, and physical—begin to contract. If we ignore this contraction for too long, it can color the way we perceive our reality, and what is very unnatural to a healthy body begins to seem natural. Because this process occurs over extended periods, as in the aging process, we often lack the awareness that it is happening until we are beyond simple fixes. With recognition, however, we can use this contraction for another purpose: to create the *in-tense(ness)* necessary to overcome our distortions in perception and regain a more wholesome perspective.

We don't have to look very far to remove the film that colors our perceptions. If we work systematically in responding to what we find in our limitations, we can perceive confrontation as a useful, often necessary, component of growth.

Consider the beginner's approach to difficult poses—even the relatively simple ones—that challenge flexibility, balance, or strength. These poses take our attention directly into areas of our body that are unfamiliar, painful, or unresponsive. This is often confronting. Stiff people have to learn how to work with pain, which is often intense, in order to remove the obstructions found in tight muscles or joints. Typically this work is associated with movement where previously no movement existed or where it was extremely limited. The weak or overly flexible have to learn how to work without overworking, to create the support or resistance necessary to bring about the subtle movement of energy in the body to build stamina or strength.

It is a common experience for both types to question why they lack movement or feeling in these areas in the first place and to wonder if there will ever come a day when it could be different. This is the beauty of the confrontation found in yoga, where opposites attract and working simultaneously with effort and non-effort is a very important lesson to learn.

With many of the *asana* that a beginner tackles for the first time, it is common to struggle with the opposing forces of particular actions found in a pose. Attempting to relax tight muscles is not easy when we are receiving a steady stream (or scream) of more demanding messages in the seemingly undecipherable language of pain. It can feel like the very resistance we experience has been protecting us from injury or overdoing something and that to surrender into this discomfort would be unwise.

Likewise, working with weak muscles to stay in a pose, to dig a little deeper, even for one more breath, seems to go against all of the yogic principles of nonviolence (*ahimsa*), and the anxiety that this can produce is real. Fatigue (mental and physical) seems to threaten our very existence, and every cell in our body is convinced that we're approaching an injury or a near-death experience.

By its very nature, though, *hatha* yoga takes us on a confrontational journey that can produce the awareness required to overcome ingrained resistance and penetrate the dense matter of our consciousness. For those with chronically tight or weak muscles, the correct practice of *asana* with conscious breathing forces the mind into a very alert state and very quickly fills the gaps typically found in a beginner's attention. This is a very important place to be. In it, we are given an opportunity to feel the power of this situation physically, to observe the dynamics of stress in an intense environment, and to overcome the mental or emotional struggle inherent in that predicament.

Of course, entering these situations in your practice requires a little preparation, and in the event of any preexisting conditions, it is beneficial and highly recommended to work with an experienced teacher who can suggest modifications to challenging poses. However, once you become familiar enough with your edge to gaze at what lies beyond it, an exterior guide will only be a distraction. Instead, you can reach inside yourself—toward your inner teacher—for guidance. That path, once mastered, prepares the understanding necessary for the more advanced practices of yoga and meditation, where, with patient, persistent effort, you strengthen your mental focus and build confidence as the initial confrontation transforms into intelligence and wisdom.

## SOFTENING

As I slowly applied this new understanding for myself, I came to see that a holistic approach to stiffness and pain had more to do with creating *softness* in the body—an openness to possibilities—and less to do with *stretching* to get somewhere other than where I currently was. It wasn't about reaching or achieving a "correct" pose. To create softness first required presence, a state in which mind and breath could meet in the container of my body, with no agenda other than to discover a new type of relating.

For me, this was a profound way to look at physical movement, especially the typical movement found in yoga practice. Even more profound was the realization that the new inner relationship I was showing up for on my mat was a perfect mirror for how to show up for the outer relationships in my life, where I was also experiencing unconscious patterns of gripping with those "problem" people in my life who seemed to make things more challenging than I thought they needed to be. If creating more intimacy with the stiff areas of my body through simple presence could create more softness, space, and connection, what would happen if I extended my experiment in softness and started a new kind of personal relationship with family and friends? When confronting interpersonal challenges, could I consciously breathe into my places of pain (stored stress) and, with each exhale, create a quality of softness that would automatically release pain? The answer was yes. All I really had to do was show up in the moment and meet others softly and as fully present as I could, with an open heart, listening to a quiet voice inside that guided me in how to be and stay present.

How we meet resistance on the mat is a beautiful reflection of how we meet resistance in life.

Our practice, both on and off the mat, is one of seeking out millimeter miracles. Those subtle shifts that take place over time, moment by moment, with presence, patience and a willingness to move in pace with our own intuition.

**Fiji McAlpine**, LEVITYoGA teacher trainee

## WHEN A GROOVE BECOMES A RUT

Patanjali's *Yoga Sutras* warn that one of the major obstacles of the mind that students face is boredom or mental laziness (*styana*). At various stages of yogic development, there is a tendency of the mind to drift away from the routine parts of the exercises; this is often the result of familiarity or mindless repetition. Some styles of yoga are more prone to this obstacle than others, especially those driven by memorized recipes or set sequences, which are often practiced over years or decades without deviation. When we observe this tendency in ourselves, when the mind wanders from the subtle experiences that are necessary to keep concentration focused and attention turned inward, we can know that our practice is suffering. It was through this realization that the seeds for developing a uniquely creative and personal style of yoga were planted in me.

As our journey toward a consistent *hatha* yoga practice overcomes the obstacles we initially encountered, we get into a rhythm, find our "groove," discover our "comfort zone," and everything flows. Then, often—without our noticing it—our groove becomes a rut. Through repetition, part of the mind goes dormant and another part of the mind takes over and breaks our "flow." The momentum we felt building inside us in terms of health, intelligence, strength, or flexibility stalls. This will often be when our practice is at risk of a long-term sabbatical, when it is easy to fall into an attitude of complacency or defeat.

Although these episodes can bring varying degrees of frustration or even desolation, it is useful to acknowledge them as part of the process and to know that during these times lies a great potential for growth. Overturning the decay of an old way of doing or seeing something lays the groundwork for what lies ahead of or within us. If our attitude toward our practice has been cultivated properly from the very beginning, we will see these occasions as moments to sharpen our attention, reassess the direction we have taken or where our focus has been led, and adjust if necessary to uncover what comes next. No matter what shows up next, can we remain calm, quiet, and alert, in a position to respond appropriately?

## RESISTANCE, SURRENDER, AND THE INTUITIVE RESPONSE

On my yoga journey, I was awakened to the truth that surrender of effort is the most efficient means to strengthen the connection I have with ground—literally, with the earth beneath that is responsible for the subtle effects of gravity. To experience that connection more intimately required awareness of how the sensations of gravity moved through me.

When movement and alignment are by-products of surrender, the flow of sensation created by muscular release creates an intuitive response in the connective tissue of our bodies. It works first by creating softness mentally when resistance to movement is present. This is usually evident when we feel some degree of discomfort in the body, such as working with tight muscles or joints. To create softness requires placing our attention into our discomfort and discovering where we have habitually contracted in reaction to what is unpleasant. Once the awareness is there, it requires patience and consistency to return to this place with the sensation of every breath, until the discomfort changes and some form of release appears. In this way, resistance becomes our inner teacher guiding us to where our attention is lacking.

This process may happen instantly, or it may take time. Yet in that moment of release, when the grip of a particular muscle on a joint or bone lets go, a sensation is generated, followed by an invitation to respond. In each yoga *asana,* inherent in its shape and form, two non-muscular processes can be used to support movement: one external, the other internal. *Gravity is the external process. Breath is the internal process.* And once movement is supported by these forces, the muscles respond, without losing the sensation generated by the release. This work is very subtle and requires alert awareness.

## LETTING GO OF GETTING "THERE"

The instructional language used by those of us who have taught in the Iyengar tradition carries a subliminal message that there is a right way and a wrong way to practice poses, and only if you follow the rules will you achieve all that yoga promises. Although I achieved mastery of many poses in that tradition—and I took some level of pride in reaching the final pose through years of following directions precisely—I came to realize how rare it was to find any instruction for what happens *after* reaching the peak of the pose. *Then what?* My back injury gave me an opportunity to work without attachment to what any final pose might look like, and I gained the insights that it's not the destination that's important—it's what you discover along the way. When working each day along the way, you never quite get "there."

If there's no importance in reaching the final pose, then what's the point? Actually, it's freedom. Detaching from the goal of reaching the final pose allows us to surrender, willfully, to what is, in any given moment. This is a powerful place to be. It was here that I discovered how to awaken intuition, and later I realized that the part of the brain responsible for intuition is the very part of the brain where yoga happens. It is where we make a connection, or union, between the hemispheres of the brain and experience a feeling of being in the zone, a state where things flow perfectly in unison. The idea of simultaneous effort and non-effort is inherently one of never truly meeting.

The physical practice of yoga is an activity that focuses on *alternating cycles of movement and stillness* as we progress deeper and closer to the ultimate pose. As the "end" of a pose approaches, going further becomes extraordinarily refined. The shape and direction of our body's movement becomes so infinitesimal as we approach the anatomical limit of a joint, muscle, or tissue that the difference between effort and non-effort is virtually imperceptible, and essentially, they become one.

## RESISTANCE AS YOUR INNER TEACHER

One of the hardest things to sell as a teacher is the fact that meeting discomfort in body and mind is an essential part of yoga. Who in their right mind would buy into that, especially a beginner? It takes a certain level of maturity and life experience to understand the value in such an idea: that inevitable in life are circumstances in which expectations fall short, obstacles appear unexpectedly, and we hit dead ends and are forced to retreat, with no one there to help.

At odds with this is a predominantly Western notion of progress being a mostly straight line, moving forward at all times, using whatever means necessary—willpower, positive thinking, intentionality—to make it happen. Anything else is perceived as failure, though the masters of any vocation or art know the contrary. To begin or renew a more intimate type of relationship with yourself requires a new attitude toward resistance: perceiving it as the gift it truly is. With that realization, you can move a little closer to a true, authentic relationship with all of who you are.

Two of the most powerful approaches to the practice of yoga in the face of resistance are patience and kindness toward yourself—the recognition and acknowledgment that where you are in this very moment is exactly where you are meant to be. No matter what circumstances took you into your current situation, especially when you are experiencing challenges or pain of some kind in your life, there is a gift hidden in the predicament—something that is there to propel you into the next phase of your life (intended or unintended), requiring an open attitude and the best possible effort, with empathy toward yourself, no matter what shows up. The experience of compassion for yourself while accepting life as it is can help you develop a childlike curiosity, free from results, about what kindness and patience can produce, leading you to discover something unknown about yourself.

As the practice of yoga develops more compassion, it also initiates a paradox that may seem counterintuitive: we learn to be brutally honest with ourselves. In most painful situations, we're working with some form of limitation, and at such points in life, there is the obvious disappointment with feeling limited in realizing our full potential in the future or with losing what we were capable of in the past. On a yoga mat, *limitation has a purpose*. It provides the resistance to truly meet yourself where you are—literally, in the present moment of yourself. And this is the moment that yoga starts, no matter what your range of motion is. In this way, resistance—resulting from limitation or from attachment to the way things were or you hoped they would be—becomes your inner teacher. It guides you to know intuitively where it is appropriate to place your attention, what types of thoughts you hold about yourself, and how to move safely and efficiently when practicing yoga. This is what helps you develop tools to work within your personal means.

When you're working in a pose and anything takes you beyond the present moment of yourself, when you are driven by anything other than gentle curiosity or intuitive invitation from your own experience, be kind to yourself—stop there and save the rest for another day. The next time you practice will provide another opportunity to reconnect with that place within yourself and see if it has changed, to see if another day brings another way to see the same thing differently. Seeing those changes and the opportunities they create to go further in your practice is very empowering, helping you to grow as a human being, mentally and physically.

Ultimately, the test for whether this approach to physical yoga is a good match for you is how well this practice supports your willingness and ability to touch discomfort softly and unveil the shadow of your existence—the part of your life where you lack or avoid connection or the subconscious or "undesirable" parts of yourself, your community, or the world you live in. Sometimes you need look no further than the relationships in your life. Is your practice of yoga supporting you to be kinder and more open toward the people close to you? Are you moving toward or away from more intimacy and connection? At its core, yoga is bonding. Yoga is union. Yoga is one.

## THE OBSTACLE OF PAIN

Every yoga practitioner experiences the obstacle of pain, so I will close this chapter by offering a suggestion for how to approach pain.

In yoga, when dealing with an injury or preexisting condition, pain is your guide. Every day should include a little movement and a little pain. Your attitude toward pain will be the key to how well you are healing. If you can see pain as a guide and respond to what you're feeling without emotion, you can create more space for your body's own natural healing forces to work. Know too that as you age, limitation becomes more common. Learning to accommodate limitation is an important aspect of overcoming suffering.

The key is to become intimate with your pain.

For the things we love, intimacy is easy—it brings us even closer to the object of our affections. It is more of a challenge to commit to intimacy with things we feel ambivalent or even hostile toward, especially things within ourselves. How do we initiate intimacy with parts of ourselves we don't like or that cause us pain physically or psychologically? The first step is showing up, with no agenda, no needs, no expectations or intentions—only presence.

In a yoga pose, what techniques can you use to be fully present and to initiate connection? What grabs your attention first when moving into a pose? All poses require physical connection to the ground, so this is a good place to start. This is where your primary connection to gravity occurs. Your relationship with gravity holds the key for nearly all movement your body is capable of, especially movement found in the practice of yoga. The parts of your body that you use for grounding are primarily the feet and hands, though many poses use other parts of the body as well, including the pelvic floor and legs; the front, side, and back of the torso; and the shoulders, neck, and head.

Meeting yourself at the floor with as much compassion, understanding, and gentleness as you can helps you discover the keys the ground holds for meeting resistance and pain in your body.

# PART 3

## *Science and Yoga Meet*

The research for this book introduced me to a large, global community of like-minded people—body workers, yogis, teachers in the human potential movement, doctors, and scientists—who share similar insights that affirm new discoveries in science. In planning the contours of this book, finding a way to translate these new paradigms onto a yoga mat appeared to me a worthy goal.

As modern science catches up to ancient wisdom, there is a more holistic view of the interrelationships found in what has, for centuries, been a mechanistic view of the body and its "separate" biological systems. Current research shows an extraordinary inner-net that weaves together what were once thought to be independent systems. In part 3, we take a look at some of these interconnections to inform our practice of yoga. We look at the "provable" science of yoga's influence on the body—specific, relevant knowledge of anatomy and physiology that is helpful for yoga practitioners to know—as well as science that shares more in common with Father Charlie's notion of grace, a phenomenon that comes "from outside the three-dimensional world we know and that gravity operates within."

Before we enter these chapters, however, let me share some valuable context from a master teacher.

## A SIMPLE STATEMENT

My very first trip to India, after I said farewell to New Zealand, was to spend a year studying at the institute of my teacher's teacher, B. K. S. Iyengar. While I had many experiences there that could find a home in this book, this one is particularly relevant to the upcoming discussion of the science of the yoga body with an orientation to the physical sense of touch.

My arrival at the Iyengar Institute in Pune coincided with a week-long celebration of B. K. S.'s seventieth birthday. It ended with his giving a four-hour talk in a yoga studio packed with students, reporters, and photographers. He spoke without interruption for three hours and then, after a very short intermission, invited audience members to ask him questions.

A young reporter from the *Times of India* asked the first question: "Why do you do yoga?"

The master had just described at great length his life in yoga, and the audience was stunned by the absurdity, the naivety of the question. At first B. K. S. appeared angry, but then his face softened.

"I like the way it makes me feel," was his answer.

He moved on to other questions, but I was left contemplating his response. It could have been the obvious interpretation: it makes him feel good, and he likes feeling good. However, what came to me years later was that he liked the way it improved his *ability to feel* into the many layers of his body and the experiences of his life—physically, emotionally, and spiritually. He liked being able to connect with the effects of what he was feeling with intimacy and intelligence and to receive guidance on how to respond appropriately.

It is a simple statement: "I like the way it makes me feel." But I invite you to consider it as a kind of touchstone as you delve into these chapters.

> The sensations of your skin and [visceral
> tissues of the] body—touch, temperature,
> pain, (and a few others)—are your mind's true
> foundation. All your other senses are merely
> added-on conveniences in comparison.
>
> **Sandra and Matthew Blakeslee**

# 6

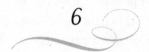

# Our Skin and Connective Tissue

Traditional science considers the skin as our one and only sensory organ of touch. Our relationship with our skin is typically superficial, but it is really one of the miracles of evolution. Our skin is an intricate organ of consummate sophistication that has developed over millions of years. It comprises three distinct layers:

- The *epidermis* is the outermost layer of skin that provides a barrier against foreign substances and trauma. It also creates our skin color and tone and contains endocrine cells called Langerhans, which act as a frontline for the immune system of the skin and other parts of the body.

- The *dermis* is the skin's thick middle layer of fibrous, elastic tissue made up of collagen and elastin. The dermis gives skin its suppleness and strength and contains sweat and sebaceous glands, nerve endings, blood vessels, connective tissue, and hair follicles.

- The *hypodermis* is the deeper subcutaneous tissue made of fat, connective tissue, nerve fibers, and blood vessels that helps insulate the body from heat and cold, provides protective padding for bones and organs, keeps the skin attached to the muscles and tendons underneath, and stores energy.[4]

As the sensory organ for touch, skin is one of the main gateways into the subconscious feeling intelligence we possess. It is also the largest organ of the body, with an area of eighteen to twenty square feet and a weight of seven to nine pounds. Sensory neurons densely enervate the skin, which has one of the highest concentrations of neurotransmitter/receptor cells outside of the brain, especially in the hands (palms, fingertips) and feet (soles, toes).

The sensory nerves of the hands and feet each have a specialized capsule on the peripheral end called a *mechanoreceptor* that physically links the nerve ending to the surrounding skin tissue. The physical sense of touch works like this: Mechanical deformations of the skin and soft tissues of the body cause a change in the shape of the capsule surrounding these nerve endings, which in turn detect this change in shape and produce a signal that is propagated to the rest of the nervous system, noting the touch's location on the skin, the amount of force, and its velocity. Other touch receptors in the skin produce additional signals in response to the object's temperature and shape, as well as the presence of chemical agents on the skin.

Sensory neurons transmit signals to the thalamus and areas of the cerebral cortex in the brain. The specific location of sensory neuron synapses in the brain determines how the touch signal is interpreted. All of our brains are similar in the broad arrangement of these sensory neurons, but research shows that "the details of the somatotopic map *characterize each individual and are determined largely by experience* [emphasis mine]."[5]

The types of touch we experience throughout our lives affect the architecture of our brains, which in turn affects our interpretation and response to different types of touch. In general, "repetitive activation of a pathway strengthens those synapses, making it easier to pass information forward."[6] Thus, the more often we experience a type of touch, the better able our brains are to interpret that information. Conversely, if there is a lack of touch, the sensory neurons will not be activated, and the synapses in that neuronal pathway will never strengthen.

For more than a century, scientists have been intrigued by the electrodermal activity of the skin and its relationship to both the sympathetic and parasympathetic nervous systems. Even more compelling is current research showing a relationship between the skin and the central nervous, immune, and endocrine systems—especially the hypothalamic-pituitary-adrenal stress axis—acting in concert to control our body's homeostasis.[7] This communication between the skin and the body's central biological and neurological systems occurs through local production and systemic release of classical hormones, neuropeptides, neurotransmitters, and biological regulators. The unique connection the skin has with the nervous and immune systems through touch is known as the neuro-immuno-cutaneous system, which displays effects through stimulation of sweat, capillary constriction or dilation, and even change in skin tone/color.[8] This common phenomenon is one that many law enforcement and military agencies use in determining if a subject is telling the truth; they measure a change in the electrical properties of a body experiencing an emotional reaction, known as the psychogalvanic reflex or galvanic skin response.[9]

## FIVE SOMATIC SENSES

Of our five physical senses, touch is unique, in that it's actually five separate somatic senses controlled by an extensive network of nerve endings and touch receptors, mostly in the skin and connective tissues. There are four main types of senses, plus one anomalous sense (not skin related, called the vestibular system, which is responsible for balance and is centered in the inner ear):[10]

- *Mechanoreception* perceives pressure (deep, gentle, and sustained), texture, vibration, stretching of skin, and the rotational movement of limbs. Its receptor cells are generally found in non-hairy skin such as the palms, lips, tongue, soles of the feet, fingertips, eyelids, and the face, as well as deeper in connective tissue along muscle, tendons, and joints.

- *Thermoreception* perceives the sensations of an object's temperature through two types of receptor cells (heat and cold) located all over the body, with the highest concentration found in the face and ears.

- *Nocireception* detects pain or stimuli that can cause damage to the body: mechanical (scrape, cut, tear, break), thermal (burn or freeze), or chemical (toxins from plants, animals, or synthetic). It's no surprise that nocireceptor cells number in the millions; are found throughout the body, not just in the skin; and perceive different types of pain, including sharp, piercing, dull, throbbing, pins and needles, tickle, and itch, to name a few.

- *Proprioception* senses the body's position and motion in space and relative to other parts of the body. There are two types of receptors: one measures stretch, which is located in muscles and tendons, indicating limb location; the other, which is located in cartilage, measures stress load and slippage in joints, indicating limb speed and direction.

Information gathered through all the somatic senses is channeled through the spinal cord and is processed in parts of the brain that produce neural maps specialized for touch and movement. These maps allow you to rapidly identify one body part from another and determine their unique locations and the physical action required to generate and coordinate optimum motion efficiently, whether you're consciously fine-tuning movement in a yoga pose or letting the autopilot of your subconscious handle low-level repetitive tasks like scratching an itch. These maps are updated constantly with new information generated by new experiences inputted through the somatic senses, developing a constantly changing sense of self.

Apart from these maps for touch and movement, even more remarkable is a third map for the visceral terrain of your inner body—your internal organs and glands. According to Sandra and Matthew Blakeslee, "This map is uniquely super-developed in the human species, and it gives us a level of access to the ebb and flow of our internal sensations unequaled anywhere else in the animal kingdom."[11] Although each of us has the ability to feel at this level, for many it remains part of the subconscious. For those of us who can sense our visceral terrain, our emotions are often the facilitators that bring this subtle awareness into the conscious realm. This is especially true around the heart—think *heavyhearted* (sadness) or *lighthearted* (joy)—and the belly—*butterflies* (anxiety/fear) and *fire in the belly* (passion/courage).

## INTERPLAY WITH THE WHOLE BEING

From its beginning, science has typically segregated and specialized parts of the body, trying to identify and categorize the unique and distinct pieces of our functional anatomy with only peripheral relationships to each other. The holistic interplay of our skin, connective tissue, muscles, bones, organs, and glands has only recently become a topic of investigation as researchers work to investigate the sizable gaps in the ability of older models of the body to fully explain how mind, emotions, and the physical systems of our bodies interrelate.

This interplay tracks with what I have discovered in my decades of yoga practice. Isolating the functions of body parts discounts the fullness of the roles they each play. Seeing the skin as the fabric of the bag of anatomical bits and pieces that we are sells it short. At its basic level, skin provides protection and a unique expression of how we meet the outside world. Dr. Bruce Lipton's research of cell membranes revealed that in single-cell organisms, the membrane itself, not the nucleus, acts as the cell's "brain."[12] (We will meet Dr. Lipton and his work again further on.) Similarly, our outer layer—the skin—has deep connections with a wide network of neural and immunological activities, as well as with the inner fascial web of connective tissue.

Recent studies show that the connective tissue system of our bodies, which begins in the dermis layer of the skin, becomes more complex and sophisticated in the hypodermis and then weaves even deeper, sharing a strong connection to the body as a whole, including bones, organs, ligaments, tendons, and muscles.[13] In fact, we are learning that connective tissue may be even more determinant in postural balance, health, and the overall architecture of our bodies than the musculo-skeletal system, contradicting the dominant view. Connective tissue may be the primary inhibitor of movement and what determines the extent of our body's stiffness or mobility.

Even more fascinating is recent research concluding that connective tissue maintains its own info-energy network that seems to communicate with other parts of fascial structures independently. This idea disputes the mainstream view that sees the nervous system as the primary conduit for motor sensory perceptions. This new model of our physical structure attributes our mobility to fascial inhibition that is both physical and psychological in nature, supporting the idea that residue from our thoughts and emotions, both positive and negative, can be stored in our connective tissue, affecting our movement deep into the fascial structure of our bodies. Although it is not yet fully understood, there is also evidence that components of connective tissue are able to detect mechanical impulses that are translated internally into cascades of biological reaction.[14]

A new science called *haptics* studies our unique sensory system of touch and its natural adaptations to strain energy and temperature sensitivity. The haptic system involves two interconnected sensory modes: *cutaneous* sensors in the skin and intradermal connective tissue and *kinesthetic* sensors in the joints, muscles, and intramuscular connective tissue.[15]

## BRINGING IT BACK TO YOGA

How do these scientific insights inform your yoga practice? Think about your experience when doing a common yoga pose like Downward-Facing Dog with your eyes closed or focused on an external point of concentration (*drishti*). Initially, the sense you have of yourself in the pose is informed by the connection your hands and feet have with the ground (or yoga mat). Both types of sensors (cutaneous and kinesthetic) tell you where your arms and legs are in space to help determine if your limbs are symmetrically placed about your center of gravity (front to back and side to side). Cutaneous sensing lets you know that you've touched the ground, with its unique texture, while kinesthetic sensing lets you know the slope or unevenness of the ground and whether it is stable enough to support your weight. Cutaneous sensing alerts you to how slippery or sticky your yoga mat is (and how to adjust as needed), and the two come together again to let you control the amount of effort needed to maintain the shape and balance in your pose.

Now, if our thoughts and emotions can influence the state of our fascial health and resilience, and if fascial health has a strong influence on movement and the biological function of our organs and endocrine glands, what type of touch—physical and mental—best affects our ability to return to a state of fluid, easeful movement, balance, and biological health? In my experience with yoga poses, how we touch the ground and how we meet the physical parts of ourselves depend on the level of intimacy we have with sensations that are produced with movement into a pose, maintaining a pose, and exiting a pose—an intimacy that is a product of touching whatever shows up, especially discomfort or pain, as softly as we can.

How we touch what shows up mentally works similarly. Can we meet the sensations we experience with empathy and sensitivity and listen to what they are trying to tell us? When we learn the language of sensation that our body uses to communicate, the body cooperates. When we practice alone, the different "minds" we possess (including those in the brain, belly, and heart—more on these later) inform our movement through the subvocal dialogue we have with our body, greatly influencing the relationships we have with each level of consciousness that we understand ourselves by (see the discussion of levels of consciousness, or *koshas*, in chapter 9).

For example, on the gross physical level, if we use the word *stretch* for our intention when encountering stiffness, that term assumes and implies a linear, two-dimensional understanding of muscular function: literally, an elongation or extension between a muscle's origin and insertion across a joint or series of joints. Until recently, this was the predominant paradigm of musculoskeletal behavior. However, if we choose a different word for our inner dialogue—*soften*—the effects are completely different. The word takes into account the nonlinear, three-dimensional nature of our body's connective tissue net, which has been found to interweave and "bind muscle fibers to muscle fibers, muscles to muscles, and muscles to bones. . . . Connective tissue binds every cell in the body to its neighbors and, arguably, the internal mechanics of each cell to the mechanical state of the body as a whole."[16]

When we awaken to this realization as yoga practitioners, our relationship to movement and the signals our bodies produce is forever changed. We begin to experience the sensations we feel through nerves *and* connective tissue jointly—as equals, in a sense, for interpreting motor function.

~

Now let's take our knowledge of skin, connective tissue, and the sense of touch to explore the places in the body that often connect us to ground on the mat: our feet and hands.

The urge to transcend gravity is quite natural to man as a spiritual being, but the desire to break loose from the vitalizing bond with the solid earth is in conflict with the law of his terrestrial existence.

**Karlfried Graf Dürckheim**

7

# Our Feet and Hands

Touch, both external and internal, gives us a sense of ourselves through acute awareness of our body. But compared to the other senses, touch's influence is hard to pinpoint. That's because tactile information enters the nervous system from every angle and is felt throughout the body at a cellular level. Identifying exactly how the neurobiology of the skin works is a bit like the old Jain parable of a group of blind men trying to collectively identify an elephant by feeling its parts—except in this case, the elephant is on the run!

The local expression and production of neuropeptides or hormones determine the skin's influence on maintaining a dynamic equilibrium in interdependent body systems that are constantly in flux. It's not that important to know exactly how this works, neuron by neuron. What's important is that the quality of our presence and ability to touch has an influence on our experience when we are touching or being touched. And as neuroscience has shown, touch can also be transferred energetically: our body maps automatically track and emulate the movements and intended movements of other people around us through a system of mirror neurons that work through observation, both *direct or indirect*.[17]

I experienced this while learning in close proximity to Shandor as he demonstrated his practice. I could *feel* things that I could not directly *see*; in this way, I came to understand the essential nature of a strong connection to ground and how powerful grounding can be.

In a yoga pose, when we use our sense of touch to feel into the ground that supports us, the activation of tactile sensory information coupled with visualization—our mind meeting the sensation we feel with a mental image—influences our experience. The two working together are more powerful than either individually.[18] Awakening the cell receptors in the hands and feet in a yoga pose that they support influences the strength or flexibility of the individual parts that are working, even as the skin's receptor cells coordinate and regulate peripheral and global homeostasis of the whole body. The key to how this works in yoga is the power of the conductivity of the body, or put another way, the lack of resistance that opens up the channels of flow toward homeostasis, toward a system-wide, dynamic balancing of all the metabolic processes of the body and mind through the parasympathetic nervous system.

Wherever we place our conscious attention, the body responds. If our mind and emotions are in equanimity and fully present to the moment, the body's autonomic activity naturally moves toward equilibrium and ease (conductivity). However, if our mind and emotions are attached to an outcome and anxious about our possibilities for "success," the body's autonomic activity naturally moves toward disequilibrium and dis-ease (resistance).

For beginners, most yoga poses connect to the ground through the feet and hands: standing poses through the feet, arm balances through the hands, and various poses that use both, like Downward-Facing Dog, Wheel, Plank (face down), or Reverse Plank (face up). Anatomically, the hands and feet are endowed with an abundance of nerve receptor cells in the skin and, less well known to many yoga students, the joints. Half of the bones found in the human body are in the hands (twenty-seven in each) and feet (twenty-six in each). Both are miracles of evolution—especially the feet in the bipedal human species. Each foot has over a hundred muscles with thirty-three articulating joints to support the entire weight of the modern upright body.

Our feet can accommodate walking, quick sprints for fleeing danger, and extended periods of long-distance (and barefoot) running, a skill anthropologists have discovered only recently that ensured the survival of our earliest human ancestors as persistence hunters.[19]

One of the two indigenous cultures still practicing this form of hunting are the Tarahumara natives of northern Mexico, who became well known in 2009 with the release of Christopher McDougall's book *Born to Run*, a remarkable story about one man's journey to reclaim his love and passion for long-distance running after injuries took both away.[20] This tale went against not only the popular thinking of the day but also what the running shoe industry in 1972 had sold the world on—the promise of a better, faster, and safer way to run. To this day, I often say, with no reservations, that McDougall's book is one of the best yoga books I've ever read, and the word *yoga* isn't mentioned once. The reason is that it clearly shows that the anatomical structure of our feet is an intricate weight-suspension system designed to naturally support the human body's static and dynamic forces of balance and movement. They are what Leonardo da Vinci considered "a masterpiece of engineering and a work of art."[21] Feet bound in running shoes, with arch support and cushioned soles whose intended function is preventing injuries, are extremely limited and create the worst possible situation for healthy functioning of the feet and, subsequently, of the knees and hips and the structural integration of the body in general.

McDougall details numerous studies going back to 1976 about the rise in runner-related injuries since the boom in popularity of air sole–cushioned running shoes. The studies are a testament to what yogis have understood for thousands of years: the bare human foot "receives a continuous stream of information about the ground and its own relationship to it (dynamic balance), while the shod foot 'sleeps' inside an unchanging environment."[22] When we press down into our feet but simultaneously lift our arches to ground ourselves, as is commonly taught in yoga, we create an unnatural grip in the musculature of the foot that chokes the sensitivity that the foot is capable of on its own. We assume, as do the designers of high-performance running shoes, that our feet have forgotten how to be feet.

When we look at the feet as part of an integrated whole—including the dynamic balancing forces of the legs, the pelvis, and the torso above—we recognize the role they play in connecting us to the true source of power and strength that the ground provides. Feet connect us to Earth physically and energetically, but it is from the center of ourselves—the belly—that we engage with what lies beneath us. (See chapter 8 for more on the belly.) The feet become conduits of connection to channel the upward effect gravity provides (levity), guiding us into poses with a sense of intimacy, balance, and ease.

When responding to gravity in standing poses, the weight on the feet should be evenly spread, front to back and side to side, by slight adjustments to the ankles or the body above, with the toes and bones of the feet remaining passive, allowing the muscles and connective tissues of the foot to respond in real time to the steady flow of feedback provided by gravity. Energetically, place your attention in the skin of the feet, as if you were trying to feel the texture of the floor or mat as intimately as possible.

The hands work in a similar way, though their evolution has not been as thorough in supporting the weight of the body. It is for this reason that, at times, in arm balance poses, it may take more effort with the muscles of the hands, wrists, and arms to respond to the intuitive call. For fully inverted poses standing on the hands, even the fingers are sometimes called into action to help establish balance. Like the feet, the hands become conduits to channel the effect that gravity provides.

When responding to gravity in arm balance poses, the weight on the hands—mainly the palms—should be evenly spread, front to back and side to side, by slight adjustments to the wrists, the arms, or the body above, with the fingers and thumbs passive until called into action as needed. Energetically, as with the feet, your attention is present in the skin of the hand.

Within the intimacy of contact we create with our feet and hands, the ground has something to share with the intuitive parts of ourselves. The information we receive from the ground through the skin is a starting point for yoga—both physically, through the influence gravity has on balance, movement, and effort, and psychologically, as we feel the influence of grounding on our emotions and the endocrine/nervous system responses they produce. As we build a more intimate relationship with ground through intelligent practice and contemplation of our experiences, the subtle body forces slowly awaken, drawing the priority of our physical attention from "working out" toward our psychological attention to "working in." As we make this shift, we move into yoga poses less through technique generated by mentally imposed muscular effort and more through surrender and the intuitive guidance that then appears—movement not so much by intention as by invitation.

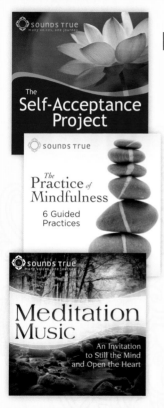
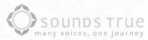

**Dear Sounds True friend,**

Since 1985, Sounds True has been sharing spiritual wisdom and resources to help people live more genuine, loving, and fulfilling lives. We hope that our programs inspire and uplift you, enabling you to bring forth your unique voice and talents for the benefit of us all.

We would like to invite you to become part of our growing online community by giving you three downloadable programs— an introduction to the treasure of authors and artists available at Sounds True! To receive these gifts, just flip this card over for details, then visit us at **SoundsTrue.com/Free** and enter your email for instant access.

With love on the journey,

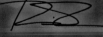

TAMI SIMON    Founder and Publisher, Sounds True

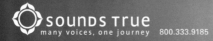
sounds true
many voices, one journey   800.333.9185

ST330

All [Hawaiian] healers know of the [life force]
energy. . . . Our ancestors and their ancestors knew
and taught of it. They called it "mana" coming from
the "na'au," or from your gut, and the "pu'uwai,"
your heart. It is as real as the ocean, as powerful
as the wind, and as infinite as the night sky.

**Paul Pearsall**

*8*

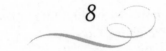

# Our Belly and Heart

The feet and hands offer the beginner to yoga a simple, familiar path
for connecting with the subtle energies present in the "feeling organ"
of skin through its relationship to gravity. However, most people come
to yoga with little or no understanding of the roles other areas in the
body play in embodying and sustaining the forces of life that animate
every cell in our body.

Throughout human history, our sentient nature has come to recognize the heart and the belly as gateways for certain emotions to
express in our psychological selves. The inseparable influence of our
emotions and thoughts on how we experience these two areas of
our physical body is well known, but few truly grasp how it works.
Even modern science has only just begun to look more seriously at the
physical implications of our psychological states. Most of us recognize
that when we're feeling at peace and balanced, our bodies feel *relaxed
and lighter*, whereas when we're anxious and out of balance, our bodies
feel *tense and heavier*. Yet our education rarely helps us see how interdependent these two states are or that we have any ability to intervene
in the process to maintain equilibrium when tension overpowers our

serenity. Both the heart and the belly have mechanisms in place to make this relationship clearer to observe, although other places in the body reflect this relationship as well.

## THE BELLY

Most of us have lost our connection to the mysterious forces at play in the abdominal region, as well as to the appearance, function, and location of the organs and glands within it. We know that this area is responsible for digestion and assimilation, but in most Western cultures, a belly is considered healthy only according to its outer appearance: flat, "cut," and firm. Good posture is supposed to be chest up, shoulders back, gut in. Emotionally, for many, the belly receives the brunt of our dysfunctional attempts to deal with negative feelings such as anger, fear, or low self-esteem.

In general, popular Western culture has placed more prominence on the head (objective intellect) and heart (individual soul) centers for discernment and transformation, while overlooking what many Eastern or so-called primitive cultures consider an essential step—the prerequisite descent into the depths of our being (lower centers), which is necessary before the ascent toward higher levels of awareness (upper centers). Our attention has moved away from the profound intelligence of the lower physical and emotional center of the body—our "guts."

However, remnants of understanding are still found in common expressions in our languages, intimating a time when we recognized the power of the lower centers. In English, to have "a gut feeling" suggests a deep understanding that often is hard to explain logically; and in the past, feelings that come from deep in our center were considered more reliable than those that came from "above": the heart or the head. Then there is someone with "guts," which implies courage and unwavering integrity.

In Japan, the word *hara* can be simply translated as "belly," but the roots of its meaning extend far beyond the physical abdomen. In Japanese culture, *hara* takes on a meaning that involves almost every aspect of life. It implies all that is considered essential to a person's character and spiritual evolvement. *Hara* is the center of the human body, but not just of the physical body. In many idiomatic Japanese expressions where the root word is found, the meanings suggest a deeper context for the term. In his book *Hara: The Vital Center of Man*, Karlfried Graf Dürckheim describes one such expression: *Hara no aru hito*.[23] It suggests not only one who possesses "center" physically, as in posture and balance, but also one who maintains balance in every way, including emotionally and mentally. This person is capable of tranquility in the face of strain, moves in and about the world with serenity, and possesses an inner elasticity that allows quick and decisive responses to any situation that arises. The *hara* is also seen as the place where the body's vital life energies collect and are expressed, whether through physical movement or energetic presence.

Hara means an understanding of the significance of the middle of the body as the foundation of an overall feeling for life.
**Karlfried Graf Dürckheim**

It is this very quality of *hara* that we look for in our yoga practice. What is referred to in Patanjali's *Yoga Sutras* as *sthira sukham* is a state of unconditional calm that is not dependent on any outward circumstances. When in it, we command heightened sensitivity and an increased readiness to meet the unexpected. Here we realize that our capacity for appropriate response in the practice of *asana* can only come from the genuine absence of tension, coupled with the correct attitude of mind and lightness of heart. Throughout the practice of yoga poses, cultivating softness in the belly helps release a subtle downward flow and sense of fluidity that can be felt there and moving down into the pelvic floor, providing an intuitive invitation to move more deeply in all poses, especially those that turn or lengthen through the waist. (This will be discussed in more detail in "Belly Consciousness" in chapter 15.)

How the belly "thinks" intuitively could be a function of what science is now calling our second brain, or the enteric nervous system, which is an extensive network of neurons embedded in the lining of our gastrointestinal tract, from esophagus to anus.[24] In addition to its handling of nearly all the digestive functions of our intestines, it is important to understand how this system of neurons intimately connects with our autonomic nervous system and, through the vagus nerve, becomes a critical component of parasympathetic control of the heart, lungs, and intestines.

The vagal channel of communication between the abdominal organs and the brain includes branches of cardiac and pulmonary ganglia, which suggests a shared relationship among these organs as well and offers a scenario in which the interrelationships are established both anatomically and energetically. The enteric system includes many of the same neurotransmitters found in the brain, including dopamine (in the intestines, it reduces peristaltic movement and maintains the inner linings of the intestinal tract; in the brain, it stimulates desire and motivation for reward response, or pleasure),[25] serotonin (in the intestines, it stimulates peristaltic movement; in the brain, it regulates mood, appetite, and sleep),[26] and acetylcholine (in the intestines, it stimulates peristaltic movement; in the brain, it regulates arousal, attention, memory, and motivation).[27]

Numerous scientific studies have shown that the voluntary control of slow breathing has a substantial positive effect on our parasympathetic response. There is multidirectional communication via vagal signals to and from the brain to quiet frontal cortical activity, as well as an inhibitory influence upon the heart and sympathetic nervous system activity and to and from the gastrointestinal tract that improves peristaltic function while strengthening immune system response in the gut.[28] (How to establish patterns of conscious breathing will be discussed in chapter 14, "Back-Body Breathing.")

> Breathing is not merely an in-drawing and out-streaming of air, but a fundamental movement of a living whole, affecting the world of the body as well as the regions of the soul and mind.
> **Karlfried Graf Dürckheim**

## THE HEART

To examine the qualities of the heart, the starting point is much easier. We have a basic understanding of the physical properties of this single, well-known organ and the role it plays in pumping blood throughout our bodies to keep us alive. On occasion, we can feel our heart beating and even hear it in moments of deep silence. However, knowledge beyond this, especially when we consider the psychological role it plays in our lives, is considerably more mystical. As a species, we have evolved with an enduring mythology about the heart's role in all matters of love. In our "heart of hearts," we know that the pulsating organ in our chests holds the energy for all our affections—love, kindness, compassion, gratitude, and more—symbolized in our cultural narrative by the familiar symmetrical heart-shaped image. But could it be that these energies of the heart that most people feel comfortable talking about, especially around Valentine's Day, have more to offer us in terms of overall health and well-being? With heart disease the number one cause of death globally for the past sixty years,[29] new branches of science (such as neurocardiology, cardio-energetics, and psychoneuroimmunology) are now looking outside the purely mechanistic view of the heart, combining the fields of cellular biology, quantum physics, modern cardiology, and ancient Eastern body-mind philosophy to better understand the heart's energetic nature and the influence the "owner" of a living heart has in sustaining and maintaining its well-being and the life of the body it occupies.[30]

In his book *The Heart's Code*, Dr. Paul Pearsall suggests that "the heart thinks, cells remember, and that both of these processes are related to an as-yet mysterious, extremely powerful, but very subtle energy with properties unlike any other known force."[31] Though he admits he is uncertain that this force exists and how it works, he thinks the mechanistic view of the heart is also uncertain, failing to acknowledge the existence of "a life force that medicine cannot yet see."[32]

Dr. Pearsall has seen that communication between the heart and the cells of the body operates on many levels: electrical, chemical, and through a force he refers to as "L" (love) info-energy, which appears to travel instantaneously and non-locally, independent of time and distance. Speaking like a true yogi, Pearsall writes:

The quantum physics principle of non-locality says that, in the minuscule buzzing quantum world of which our body's cells are a part, there are no barriers, time is relative . . . , that mass, energy, and information are one and the same, that objects once connected forever retain the info-energetic memory of that connection, and [that] the separateness of any kind in the world, human or otherwise, is mere illusion.[33]

I sense the day will arrive when researchers will establish the connections between the subtle energies of the heart, brain, and gut—but not through the scientific methods of mind alone. It will happen in the realms where yoga has understood this principle for thousands of years—through the direct experience of movement, mind, and breath. Could it be that when more scientists adopt a personal practice of yoga and meditation—or any other body-mind practice that awakens the knowledge of the body's healing power within—they will have firsthand experience to report (as opposed to secondhand data to interpret) how our psychology and physiology merge in the subtle body? It seems to be only a matter of time.

The brain and heart each possess mutually dependent "minds" that control aspects of the other. Both have an influence on how "L" info-energy is transmitted and received, based on their respective neurological states (excitation/anxiety or inhibition/relaxation) and unique natures. The brain has a split personality, with its dominant, primitive, and emotionally immature aspect often overriding responses from its more recently evolved thinking and intuitive centers—or over any emotional intelligence expressed from the heart or gut. Pearsall describes the brain as "the ultimate 'type A' . . . always in a hurry." The heart is more of a type B—more gentle, relaxed, and subtle. According to Pearsall, "The brain seems to want to 'have a blast' while the heart needs to 'have a bond.'"[34]

The heart has its reasons which reason does not understand.
**Blaise Pascal**

Pearsall cites research on the subtle energy connection and human consciousness conducted for over twenty years at the Engineering Anomalies Research Lab at Princeton University. From this and his own research of heart transplant patients, he identifies the following five simple qualities and principles of the heart that provide statistically relevant evidence of the possibility of nonphysical heart "L" info-energy. As a student of yoga, I found this familiar territory, similar to the heartful practices that welcome the nonphysical qualities of the subtle body, especially those of lightheartedness and levity; my parallel comments in italics follow Pearsall's words.

- **BE PATIENT** — the brain's way is to "just do it"; the heart's way is to "let it be." *In yoga, this quality of the heart that informs a state of being is known as* kshama, *or patience, and is one of the five* yamas *in Patanjali's* Yoga Sutras.

- **BE CONNECTED** — try to "unite" more than "control"; and to do "our thing" rather than "your own thing"; the energy of bonding—remember the uniquely powerful "loving bond" connection and the impact of that shared energy signature on other persons, places, and things. *This state of being is the primary goal and the essential definition of the word* yoga *(union).*

- **BE PLEASANT** — the brain tends to be defensive, negative, and prone to hostility, but the heart's nature is to be agreeable, congenial, and harmonious. To connect with our heart, we have to be more like our heart. *In yoga, this quality of the heart is known as* santosa, *a state of serene contentment, and is one of the five* niyamas *in Patanjali's* Yoga Sutras.

- **BE HUMBLE** — realize that your idea of "self" is your brain's illusion of separateness. We are all connected and mutually dependent as participants in a universal system. *In the most important way, being humble is about truthfulness, or satya, another of the ten yamas, where we understand our true, universal nature, which is not separate from others—we are not superior or inferior to anyone.*

- **BE GENTLE** — take it easy, take your time, and take what comes. Using our heart to moderate and instruct the brilliant brain with its wisdom, we have to start learning to want what we have instead trying to have what we want. *This state comes from a respect and deep kindness toward ourselves, others, and all things; it is the primary energy needed to open and create flow in the central channel of our subtle body, known as* sushumna.[35]

During the practice of yoga, surrendering and softening into the space around the heart creates receptivity to the energies the heart generates, receives, holds, or transmits. Mentally imposed muscular effort around the heart, however, only serves to weaken its capabilities and what lies within it. Understanding how to breathe efficiently is another cornerstone for awakening to the lightness in spirit that the heart contains. Opening space around the heart through surrender and breath provides buoyancy for the heart's energy to naturally expand. Like the gut, the heart responds to stillness and the absence of effort; when combined with the knowledge of correct posture and a consciously relaxed belly, it brings a shift in presence. (Opening to the energies of the heart during your yoga practice will be discussed in more detail in "Chest Dropping" in chapter 15.)

You may consider yourself an individual, but . . . you are in truth a cooperative community of approximately fifty trillion single-celled citizens. Almost all of the cells that make up your body are amoeba-like, individual organisms that have evolved a cooperative strategy for their mutual survival. [Basically] human beings are simply the consequence of "collective amoebic consciousness."

**Bruce Lipton**

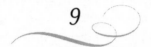

# 9

# *Into the Subtle Worlds*

Until yoga became firmly embedded in my life, the simplistic, mechanistic view of how my body worked was sufficient: the brain was the captain, the heart was second mate, and everything else—the muscles, the bones, and the only other organs I vaguely had a sense of (lungs, stomach, bladder, anus, genitals, though not necessarily in that order)—were the soldiers. The soldiers took orders from the captain when it came to solving problems or getting stuff done and from the second mate when situations of life, death, or love arose that the brain was unwilling or unable to deal with. Talking about energy, consciousness, or anything to do with the subconscious mind was inconceivable, even contemptible. I trusted entirely my brain's abilities to overcome any problem, especially when my heart was broken. When that didn't work, I was at a loss.

But once I fully entered yoga, my life experiences gradually helped me see the limited view I had of my mind, heart, and soul, and I was ready to receive more of what yoga had to offer, especially in the realms of the subconscious parts of myself—the *koshas*—where the physical and psychological connect. Yoga offered me mastery over the fluctuations of my busy mind; freedom from trying to resolve every problem I had or thought I might someday have; and an alternative view of mental and emotional awareness that was powerful, focused, and clear.

As with everything that came before, I was driven to learn it "all" in as short a time as possible. This was essentially paradoxical: I was trying to use an untrained mind to learn more about the mind. It took me years to get over this hump. But I later realized it hadn't been a climb; the hump just slowly disappeared over time. I eventually came to know what I hadn't known at the start—*yoga teaches us yoga*. That knowledge comes as we gain experience through movement, study, and connection to others. We learn from teachers and fellow students and, if we are called to teach, from our students' questions. Amazingly, no prerequisites are necessary to begin practicing yoga. The practice always starts where you are.

## THE *KOSHAS*

What are the *koshas*? In very simplistic terms, yoga philosophy defines a human "being" (noun) within five body states of "being" (verb) human. Each of us has five bodies made of increasingly finer grades of energy and consciousness; the following is summarized from various translations of a classical yoga text called the *Taittiriya Upanishad*:

- Human beings consist of a material body, or anatomical sheath, built from the food they eat. Those who care for this body are nourished by the universe itself.

- Inside this is another body made of life energy. It fills the physical body and takes its shape. Those who treat this vital force as divine experience excellent health and longevity, because this energy is the source of physical life.

- Within the vital force is yet another body, this one made of thought or mental energy. It fills the two denser bodies and has the same shape. Those who understand and control the mental body are no longer afflicted with fear.

- Deeper still lies another body made up of intellect. It permeates the three denser bodies and assumes the same form. Those who establish their awareness here free themselves from unhealthy thoughts and actions, and develop the self-control necessary to achieve their goals.

- Hidden inside is yet a subtler body, composed of pure joy and spirit. It pervades the other bodies and shares the same shape. It is experienced as happiness, delight, and bliss.

Like Russian matryoshka nesting dolls, these five bodies, also known as *sheaths* or *fields*, each fit within the next (see figure 1 on page 80). Only the densest of these is made of matter as we know it; the other four are energy states invisible to the physical eye, though we can easily sense their presence inside us when we pay close attention. Since the inner bodies are the source of our well-being during life and in many ancient Indian texts are considered the vehicles we travel in after death, the original yogis developed specific exercises to strengthen and tone each sheath in turn. For example:

- As we learn to still or quiet disruptions and clear stagnation in our anatomical sheath (*annamaya kosha*) through the practice of physical yoga, our awareness of our life energy sheath (*pranamaya kosha*) increases and is more readily accessible.

- As we learn to still or quiet disruptions and clear stagnation in our life energy sheath (*pranamaya kosha*) through breathing practices (*pranayama*) and relaxation exercises (*yoga nidra*), our awareness of our mental sheath (*manomaya kosha*) increases and is more readily accessible.

- As we learn to still or quiet disruptions and clear stagnation in our mental energy sheath (*manomaya kosha*) through withdrawal of the senses (*pratyahara*) and the first step of meditation concentrated on a fixed object or point (*dharana*), our awareness of our intellect field (*vijnanamaya kosha*) increases and is more accessible.

- As we learn to still or quiet disruptions and clear stagnation in our intellect field (*vijnanamaya kosha*) through the final step of meditation (*dhyana*), we realize "fluid, moment-to-moment awareness" and the ultimate awareness of our spirit or bliss field (*anandamaya kosha*). Here, "subject and object unite in a state of no-mind and no-time," individuality and universality merge, and what remains is pure awareness and expansive presence in totality.[36]

When I first learned these principles of consciousness in India, the vocabulary was foreign to me, even though the teachers spoke English;

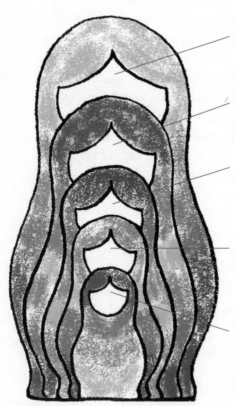

**ANATOMICAL SHEATH (*Annamaya*)**
Outmost gross physical body: bone, tissue, organs, fluids, cells.

**LIFE ENERGY SHEATH (*Pranamaya*)**
Subtle energy source of sensations or "winds" (*vayus*) that support our biological processes.

**MENTAL SHEATH (*Manomaya*)**
Thought energy that permeates and influences the previous two sheaths and includes sensory and motor activities directed from the brain and the central nervous system.

**INTELLECT FIELD (*Vijnanamaya*)**
Discerning and intuitive awareness that permeates and influences the previous three sheaths and includes self-awareness and discretion.

**BLISS/SPIRIT FIELD (*Anandamaya*)**
Innermost awareness of Higher Self where spirit and matter embrace; produces pure joy experienced as happiness, delight, and bliss beyond matter or thought.

**FIGURE 1** The five sheaths of human being: *pancha koshas*

my logical brain struggled to make sense of it all. Over the next twenty years, through regular visits to my yoga mat in the mornings, I gradually developed a sense of each sheath and how to recognize and reside in each, even if just momentarily. The effects of the physical practice of yoga have produced energetic and mental experiences of each layer that had no precedent for me before I experienced them; it was only through study and conversations with other teachers that I deciphered the language my body was using to communicate between the subconscious and the conscious. Based on those experiences and the research that follows, I believe yogic techniques are available that approximate what modern science is beginning to find and that the conscious and subconscious can communicate back and forth, with each recognizing the effects of this dialogue.

## NEW SCIENCE CATCHES UP

In recent years, scientific frontiers in neurobiology, neurocardiology, neuroendocrinology, and psychoneuroimmunology have gradually encroached upon the domains of these age-old concepts, and the language from both sides now seems more fluent and congruent. I consider myself a novice of scientific intellectual inquiry and acknowledge that my strengths lie elsewhere, particularly in the intuitive sensitivities and insights I have found from somatic experiences on my yoga mat. Yet as luck would have it, the science books I reference in this chapter were written with readers like me in mind, with easy-to-follow descriptions of complex relationships that, like yoga, are woven together with paradox and with many describing insights that cannot be measured. Yet self-evident truths are found within all of them. This is something Father Charlie often talked about in his lectures:

> So, how can the truth ever be known? The answer is always only through what the Buddha called your heart-mind. When you find that self-evident truth, there will be no need to confirm it, nor to convince others that what is true for you is also true for them. [May you break] free from any doctrine that keeps you from knowing what was always yours to know.[37]

Before I read these "science for the un-scienced" books, much of what I knew about the brain and nervous system was based on information learned in school decades ago—information that had not weathered the test of time well. The new language the writers of these books used to describe intricate concepts miraculously arrived in my life just in time for me to complete these chapters.

## LEARNING FROM CELLS

In his book *The Biology of Belief,* Dr. Bruce Lipton, whom we first met in our discussion of the senses, describes having a "scientific epiphany" that shattered his beliefs about the nature of life and human cells. While reviewing research he had done on the mechanisms cells use to control their physiology and behavior, he suddenly realized that a cell's life is fundamentally controlled by its *environment*—physically and energetically—with only a small contribution from its *genes*.[38] This insight flew in the face of the dogma of the day, known as genetic determinism—the belief that our lives are determined by our genes—which was, and for some continues to be, the only scientifically accepted belief.

From these insights evolved two new fields of science: *signal transduction,* which "recognizes that the fate and behavior of an organism [are] directly linked to its perception of the environment"—meaning that the character of our life is based on how we perceive it[39]—and *epigenetics,* the root words of which mean "control above genetics," or as Lipton puts it, "the science of how environmental signals select, modify, and regulate gene activity."[40] Lipton maintains that our genes' activity changes in response to our experiences, which means that our perceptions shape our biology.

Our body's inner "galaxy" is composed of forty to fifty *trillion* cells. The basic parts of a typical cell are the outer lining (membrane); a structural network of thin fibers (cytoskeleton), which helps with shape, division, and movement; the jellylike interior fluid (cytoplasm); the central core matter (nucleus), which protects DNA and directs cellular metabolism; and all the rest—little, floaty "bits" in the cytoplasm (such as organelles and Golgi apparatus), moving about, performing critical, life-dependent jobs such as creating and transporting proteins, assimilating food into energy, and eliminating waste.

Until now, the assumption was that the nucleus is the "brain" of the cell, based on the 1953 discovery of chromosomes and DNA. The theory of the primacy of DNA implies that DNA controls your life and that you cannot influence your DNA. But it's not that cut and dried. Lipton's cell experiments showed that if the cell's nucleus and its DNA-containing material are removed, the cell does not immediately die; though they could not divide or reproduce, the "brainless" cells he studied continued to live, eating, excreting, respiring, moving, and even communicating with other cells and responding to the environment.

So, if the nucleus is not the brain, or at least not all of it, where in this little bubble of goo is the brain? Dr. Lipton found clues, hidden in earlier research, implying that a cell's extremely thin outer membrane is much more sophisticated and complex than it first appeared and was the most likely candidate. Through studies on one of the most primitive single-cell organisms on Earth—the prokaryote, which exists with no nucleus, only a membrane and cytoplasm—Lipton recognized that these simple cells could carry out basic physiologic processes in ways similar to more complex, "sentient" cells.

Lipton found that, like the organ of skin that covers our human body, the outer skin of the cell body is a three-layered sheath, with chemical and electromagnetic channels and gates that attract beneficial substances and repel harmful ones. The cell membrane's sense of touch is similar in many ways to our skin's sense of touch, capable of feeling what it encounters chemically and energetically and responding appropriately. The membrane can physically alter its shape to adapt itself as needed and, like our body's skin, regenerate itself on a regular basis.

This idea is interesting for the practice of yoga because of the membrane's capacity to "read" energy fields, especially those broadcast continuously from the heart that reach into every cell in the body. If where we consciously place our emotional attention can affect the heart's physical and energetic rhythms, and if the energy fields of our beating heart can reach into the depths of our cellular biology, *and* if what Dr. Lipton is saying is true—that cell membranes are sensitive to environment forces, including thoughts—then we can begin to see potential in our growing awareness of the subtle body through yoga. Thus, we arrive at a powerful way to rewire our genetic program beyond just wishful thinking.

We in the West have taken for granted that there's only one brain that controls the entire nervous system in all its dimensions. As I continued my research for this book, I began to realize how simple it would have been for yogis in ancient times to have only one "brain's" mind to still the fluctuations of! But they well understood that the picture is so much vaster and more complex than that—it boggles all of my "minds," in a good way. Finally, science is starting to recognize this as well.

How can this new understanding of our "brains"—existing in the head, the heart, the gut, and even at the cellular level—be applied to help us get a clearer picture of the collective "minds" our body contains? Let me present a few more ideas from my research, hopefully in a more yogicly tempered, less scientifically intense vocabulary than I encountered in my reading.

In documenting his discoveries and insights about cell membranes, Lipton was self-aware in the way his insights came to him—through pure coincidence. He saw for the first time while revisiting old notes the remarkable similarities between the internal functions and behavior of molecules inside the cell membrane and those of liquid crystals inside digital watch faces and laptop computer screens, simply because he intuitively reached for a publication close by that had nothing to do with biology: a computer manual. From that moment on, he saw the cell membrane as a "liquid crystal semi-conductor with gates and channels," and he later found the analogy made his challenging conclusions about cells a little easier for people to swallow.[41] If a cell is like a programmable chip, then *of course* it could be influenced by signals coming from outside itself.

## LIFE FORCES AT WORK

Over the past fifty years, numerous scientific studies have consistently demonstrated that invisible forces such as electromagnetic frequencies can influence biological processes, and even that these forces communicate more efficiently than physical signals.[42] Our earliest yoga ancestors learned how to create a flow of life-force energy through their subtle bodies, and they taught these skills to their students down through the ages. If I, as a yoga practitioner, can learn to do this for myself, it is clear to me that this is where the crossover occurs: If in practice, we merge the physical with the subtle, we can let go of "trying" to heal ourselves. We don't need to understand all the intricate processes of the multitrillion-member community of cell organisms that we are. Instead, we can come to understand through our practice that the deep calm that yoga produces is a by-product of our connection to ground and that the mind in our heart-belly-brain centers knows what to do from there. Our body (including every cell) and all of our "minds" understand that we are all one.

Learning how to create this state of flow requires a closer examination of this expanded nature of mind, starting with its relationship to our brain and nervous system.

## THE NERVOUS SYSTEM

As solitary single-cell organisms evolved, the "signal" molecules they released to regulate their own physiologic behavior also influenced the behavior of other organisms. Over millions of years, this dispersed community of solitary cells figured out that cell survival improved if they bonded together and shared their "awareness" to coordinate behavior. As the size and functional complexity of these organisms increased, a new type of cell was required to create community-based control to arbitrate between the needs of individual cells and the multicellular organism as a whole. This was the beginning of our central nervous system; indeed, many of our own signal molecules, such as hormones and neuropeptides, came from our single-cell ancestors. The central processor of our nerve network is the brain, which coordinates signal molecule communication within the community of cells.[43] The brain took on the job of controlling the behavior of the cells.

As the complexity of the human organism increased, the brain developed specialized departments to manage its authority over the collective community's biological needs. Because survival was the primary need, some departments were responsible for "attacking" (eating) or for "escaping" (from being eaten). Today we call this department the limbic system, or the paleomammalian cortex. The development of this system was a major evolutionary advance and formed a majority share of our earliest humanoid ancestors' brains, which converted chemically induced signals into sensations—emotions (the sensations of "e"nergy in motion)—to alert the cellular community that action was needed. But it's a two-way street: the conscious mind can also produce emotions in addition to reading them, thereby making its own imprint on the nervous system.[44]

Neuroscientist Dr. Candace Pert also discovered that our mind is not focused in the head but is dispersed throughout the body. Lipton describes how in her work, Dr. Pert was able to show that our "emotions [are] not only derived through a feedback of the body's environmental information" but also through self-consciousness, "the mind can use the brain to generate 'molecules of emotion' and override the system."[45]

## REPROGRAMMING THE SUBCONSCIOUS THROUGH YOGA

One of many reasons yoga is so powerful a tool for balancing both our minds and emotions is that it has the ability to reprogram the subconscious part of our brain through conscious effort. The consistent practice of yoga provides increased intimacy with and sensitivity to subtle sensations, which is half the battle in overcoming subconscious programming. If we can feel it, we can choose to show up for it when we notice it.

To show up for the sensation, no matter what it is, means to stay present with it, not rush to change or fix it. With conscious breathing as a start, see if the sensation changes on its own in accordance with a slower rhythm of breath. Also, with each cycle of breath, you can see whether the intuitive part of your mind in places such as the brain, the heart, or the gut provides you with guidance, inviting you to move physically (with your body) or psychic-emotionally (with a change in mind, attitude, or heart). As you will see farther along, when you change the frequency of your brain wave activity to a calmer and more self-aware rhythm through regular yoga practice, you can reboot your subconscious programming through subvocal messaging or intentional visualization to reprogram your mind.

Understanding how this works makes us even more sensitive to events that push our buttons. It also helps us see how quickly the feeling center of a particular emotion causes immediate contraction of flow, or "stiff energy." If a particular limbic reaction is unwelcome and not addressed, the same plasticity of our subconscious mind to create positive change can have the opposite effect, with unintended consequences, where unconscious displays of "negative" emotions derail the functioning of an otherwise healthy body.

Another evolutionary efficiency of the subconscious mind takes the form of what Lipton calls "fundamental reflex behaviors."[46] The subconscious mind is primarily a repository of stimulus response tapes derived from both our genes and our learned experiences. The subconscious mind is fundamentally habitual. The part of the mind where buttons get pushed—where small triggers release suppressed traumatic memories or emotions out of proportion to present events—is a stored stimulus response behavior pattern, which often develops before the age of six, though it also includes repeated adult experiences. Subconscious by definition, this pattern is not usually subject to conscious control.

We are so good at creating these patterns that we can even fashion them from other people's perceptions, embedding their beliefs in our own subconscious minds—whether or not their perceptions are helpful to us or reflect reality. If what we come to learn from a teacher, a book, or an ad is based on misperceptions or on perceptions that differ from our own direct experience, they are at best equivocal and open to being either true or false. Consequently, these controlling perceptions upon which we base our behaviors would be more accurately defined as beliefs. And just as perceptions control biology, so do beliefs.

Our conscious mind is the creative part where our personality "lives," where we manifest intentions and hold the hopes and ambitions for our lives. It is the breeding ground for positive thinking. Unfortunately, trying to create lasting change in this part of the mind with affirmations is like sitting in a sailboat on a windless day and blowing as hard as you can into the sail: a lot of effort but minimal results. Writes Lipton, "When it comes to sheer neurological processing abilities, the subconscious mind is more than a million times more powerful than the conscious mind."[47] Neuroscience has established that our conscious mind is operating only about 5 percent of the time, while programs running in the subconscious mind determine 95 percent or more of our life experiences. The conscious mind can override a subconscious preprogrammed behavior, but only when the conscious mind is self-reflective and present. The moment the conscious mind stops paying attention, the subconscious program takes over.

## CREATING THE FLOW STATE

With a basic understanding now of how subconscious programming works, let's look at how the practice of yoga can help us create a state of mind that is conducive to healing. Can we find through physical practices—such as a flowing series of yoga poses—the necessary "flow" state of mind that makes the limiting aspects of the subconscious mind more vulnerable to reprogramming? And through consistent practice, can we move our creative consciousness toward momentary peaks of insight while in the heightened state of being "in the zone"?

To understand how we can do this, we need a basic understanding of neural brain activity and how it is identified. Using an electroencephalogram (EEG) monitor with small sensors placed on the scalp, scientists can measure brain activity (that is, the intensity of our thinking and emoting) through the synchronized electrical pulses that the community of brain neurons uses to communicate among themselves. Each pulse reaches a certain height (amplitude) that can be measured above and below (peak and trough) its steady (undisturbed) state. The pulse's frequency (pulse cycles per second) and bandwidth (amount of info-energy) form brain waves, corresponding to various levels of neural activity and indicating levels of consciousness.

EEG is a generalized assessment, like an average scene one would expect to find among a diverse community of neuro-activists: different parts of the brain work at different rhythms, intensities, and sometimes with different objectives, and they always change over time. There are widespread beliefs about which mind states brain waves correspond to, and mystery surrounds the recently discovered gamma wave. As with the mysteries one finds in yoga, this is not the territory for linear thinking with well-defined edges. Just look at the images in figure 2, showing the chaotic characteristics of each type of wave.

It is well known that during the "flow" state, the prefrontal cortex goes quiet, our conscious sense of self loosens its grip, and we feel more connected to the now of the moment, with heightened intuition and memory; we are fully present with whatever activity we're engaged in. The sense of time fades away, as do distractions. Psychologists refer to "flow" as a state in which brain wave activity slows down to a lower frequency, known as *theta* (4 to 8 hertz). This state comes naturally in children ages two through six, which makes sense. During this time, a kid's brain is developing; processing vast quantities of information like a sponge; soaking up learned behaviors, beliefs, and attitudes, mostly from parents or siblings; and stowing them away as synaptic pathways in the subconscious.[48] Theta frequencies are also the ones hypnotherapists elicit during treatments, when a patient's brain activity is more "programmable" and receptive.

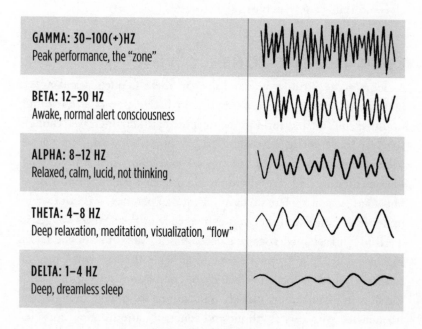

**GAMMA: 30–100(+)HZ**
Peak performance, the "zone"

**BETA: 12–30 HZ**
Awake, normal alert consciousness

**ALPHA: 8–12 HZ**
Relaxed, calm, lucid, not thinking

**THETA: 4–8 HZ**
Deep relaxation, meditation, visualization, "flow"

**DELTA: 1–4 HZ**
Deep, dreamless sleep

**FIGURE 2** Brain waves

For thousands of years, the same thing has happened in yoga, using relatively simple practices: slow, soft, conscious breathing synchronized with slow, continuous movement, linking poses one after the other, with the mind focused on coordinating movement with breath. For yogis, our neurobiological feedback system monitors the flow of inner sensation throughout the body as we move, as well as the reactions this creates for us physically and psychologically. (For more on how this is done, see chapter 16.)

With regular practice, the conscious control center of the mind is inhibited, and the subconscious mind is accessed. Well-documented scientific studies show that the brain is a plastic medium, always in a state of change, adding or subtracting synaptic couplings either electrically or chemically, and influenced by every thought we generate. As with the muscles in the body, when we exercise the brain, it gets stronger and more resilient; when we don't, it gets weaker and atrophies. What yoga brings about is easy access to the *right side* of the brain: "The territory where sensory perception, emotional acuity, imagination, dreaming, holistic thinking, creativity, and mystical experience all comfortably and synergistically coexist."[49]

## LOVE AND THE ZONE

As more access to flow is established in theta frequency and as we make peace with the self-limiting or destructive aspects of our mind, intuitive abilities and intimacy with spirit naturally increase. Though scientists have yet to determine exactly how this works, they have been able to track changes in brain wave activity when studying lifelong meditators and recently found the higher-frequency brain wave known as *gamma*.[50] Here we have yet another paradox: it is not easy to understand how the slower, lower frequency of theta waves we generate through sustained yoga practice could possibly link to the faster, higher frequency of gamma waves. Well here's the key: when meditators were asked to focus on feelings of compassion during the study, the shift in brain activity quickly transitioned from theta into gamma frequencies, with very rhythmic and coherent patterns. Now consider the psychological qualities of compassion—feeling love and empathy toward all, including ourselves and all that is. Compassion expands the boundaries of our individual egos and encompasses a worldview much larger than what our smaller self is capable of.

Gamma waves have also been discovered in elite athletes. Studies have shown that when athletes speak about being in the zone, their brains also produce the gamma state.[51] In this case, it makes sense, as we could conclude that the love top athletes have for what they do, especially when they are fully engaged in doing it, produces a similar effect as in those meditating on compassion—or, in effect, love. For both groups, gamma becomes a natural state of consciousness.

The gamma frequency corresponds to a state of peak performance. Its benefits include the following:

- Memory improves, with exceptionally vivid and rapid recall.

- Sensory perception increases, with all seven senses heightened: food tastes better, vision and hearing sharpen, sense of smell and touch become more powerful, intuition is more accessible, and humor becomes more spontaneous and lighthearted. (For more on this, see chapter 10.)

- Mental focus and processing speeds increase, with greater range and sensitivity.

- Emotional temperaments are naturally happier, calmer, and more at peace.

- Powers of creativity, intuition, and visualization expand.

- Spontaneous feelings of compassion, gratitude, love, and connection with all creation multiply.[52]

I came across one possible explanation for how theta frequencies morph into gamma in the book *Your Sixth Sense* by psychotherapist and author Belleruth Naparstek. In it, she described her process of solving this mystery for herself, consistent with the ideas we are discussing here:

Meditating on the heart, deliberately and consciously generating and holding feelings of love, gratitude, compassion and empathy produces the entrainment of heart and brain. . . . The heart frequency then drives the entire system, entraining the non-linear biological oscillators in the brain stem, intestines, vascular system, and other areas to follow suit in one coherent internal rhythm pattern of [very] low-frequency, amplified peace [below .1 HZ and significantly lower than theta or delta]. Heartfelt emotions of love and gratitude are what rule this powerful engine.[53]

As we have learned, the wave activity of our brain moves at various frequencies with unique attributes. When there is coherence of wavelengths between the brain and the heart, something magical happens. Our sense of self and the boundaries of the ego expand. As Naparstek describes it,

At the psychological level, we can say that when we open our hearts, boundaries dissolve. The ego expands and encompasses more than just the self. The I-thou distinctions, the line between self and non-self, disappears. It is no longer a matter of you and me. I become you and you become me. My energetic field opens, expands, and intersects with yours, and our realities merge. Or, if I carry it further, I merge with my family, my country, my species, with all creation, with the entire universe.[54]

With what I'm sure was the same sense of excitement and insight I experienced when reading her book, Naparstek describes finding *Stalking the Wild Pendulum* by Itzhak Bentov, who proposed, like other quantum thinkers, that all "apparently solid matter is nothing but vibration, and . . . [subatomic] particles turn out to be nothing but wave packets."[55]

Bentov described in simple terms how everything in the universe at the quantum level operates much like a pendulum. The momentary pauses at each peak of the pendulum's movement interrupt, for a nanosecond, its adherence to clock time. Here, time "stops," and in quantum physics, this escape from time opens the door to the infinite, beyond time and space. As Naparstek confirmed about Bentov's work,

> Pendulums have some remarkable features at their still points, as does anything that is at absolute rest. Between the time a pendulum has come to a full stop and the point at which it starts on its return trip, it traverses a "zero-point," where all bets are off regarding the causal relationship between time and space. At those two still points, the pendulum becomes, for a very short period of time, "nonmaterial," and expands into space at infinite velocity. Thanks to [Albert Einstein's] relativity theory, this is a mathematical certainty.[56]

"In fact," Bentov writes, "we may say that the two contrasting concepts of movement and rest become reconciled in the absolute [infinity]."[57]

Naparstek discovered that our body's electromagnetic rhythm as a whole is oscillating up and down at an average rate of 7 hertz, which means that, like the pendulum, our body's various systems of energetic pulsation arrive at a resting state a minimum of fourteen times every second. In these micro-moments, the collection of micro-particles or waves that our bodies are "expand at a very high speed through subjective time in objective space."[58] During the state of heart-mind-body coherence, the oscillations at the still points transform to match and resonate with the super-high frequency, super-low amplitude found in what Naparstek describes as "the perfectly calm, still surface of the infinite sea of pure consciousness."[59]

Of course, we have no conscious awareness of this phenomenon— of literally moving back and forth between the infinite of the quantum world and the three-dimensional world in which we physically operate—as its frequency is too quick and minuscule for our limited senses to perceive. But through the coherence created when we are in the zone—like the meditator, the athlete, or even when we fall in love—we get a sense that time stands still, and we subatomically merge or bond with the activity or environment in which we find ourselves.

In both states—in the zone and in the flow—the brain releases a cascade of biochemistry: norepinephrine, dopamine, anandamide, endorphins, and serotonin, which are all pleasure-inducing, performance-enhancing chemicals with similar benefits. Both norepinephrine and dopamine amp up focus, boost imaginative possibilities, and help us gather more information, while also lowering the brain's signal-to-noise ratios and increasing pattern recognition—our ability to link ideas in new ways. Anandamide, whose name, interestingly, was derived from the Sanskrit word *ananda* ("bliss"), is a natural pain-relieving compound that helps reduce anxiety and "increases lateral thinking—meaning it expands the size of the database searched by the pattern recognition system."[60] Endorphins also decrease feelings of pain and stress, boost feelings of euphoria, help modulate appetite, stimulate the release of sex hormones, and enhance our immune response.[61] Serotonin contributes to feelings of well-being and happiness; helps regulate our body's sleep-wake cycles, internal clock, bowel function, and appetite; and appears to regulate sexual function.[62]

Taken together, the knowledge of the neurochemical, neuroelectrical, and neurobiological plasticity in brain and nervous system function provides us with an exceptional opportunity to create the necessary conditions for restructuring our subconscious behaviors, by establishing regular states of flow and, through conscious effort, creating mental-emotional imagery and signals that provide access to the zone and let the body's inherent wisdom do the rest. Through the practice of yoga, we have the ability to consciously create calm, intimacy, and connection to ground and the subtle sensations of energy information that pass into, through, and around us. From there, we can surrender into the fact that our body and mind together understand that they are one. This is the experience the regular practice of yoga promises, as well as the new awareness yoga helps us develop with breathing. Each peak of our inhale and each trough of our exhale creates the same kind of momentary pause in time, which in turn gives us a very subtle sense of space—within and without—that we now know is infinite. At each moment between effort and non-effort, a similar space opens and time disappears. Every cycle of breath we take consciously and every oscillation between effort and non-effort we make while maintaining structure or firmness in a yoga pose—those very short periods when the waves are in coherence—remind us of our connection to the infinite. This is the zone of athletes, yogis, meditators, artists, and anyone seeking intimacy with intuition and the spark of creativity.

~

In this chapter, I have given you several different entry points to the merging of ancient and modern science as it pertains to the mind and body states that yoga practice can create. I invite you to remain open to further parallels as modern science and your own practice continue to progress.

I close this chapter with a story to illustrate what can happen at the point of stillness before the pendulum swings.

## UNFORESEEN LESSONS FROM SITTING STILL

Following my time in India with Iyengar, I had the opportunity to do something completely different: I attended a retreat at the home of S. N. Goenka, the influential teacher of Vipassana meditation from Burma who has been acknowledged for reintroducing the practice back into India. The difference between the two forms of practice—the former involving physical movement and the latter, physical stillness—could not have been more stark, and I was challenged to my core. But the discoveries I made became foundational to the approach to yoga I describe in this book. They were hard-won lessons in energetic movement through the subtle body, and the intimate connection between body and mind.

The program was ten, very full twelve-hour days spent sitting—with no talking, no music, no reading, no writing, no killing (even mosquitos), nothing that would stimulate mental activity, including napping (to avoid the mental activity of dreams). There was no kind of movement (not even fidgeting) during the sessions or in between (not even yoga).

Communication with other students—eye contact, gestures, or any type of sign language—was also to be avoided. After twelve months of consistent yoga practice with Iyengar, I felt physically prepared for the rigor of it. Mentally, though, I wasn't so sure.

On the first day, my mind was relatively quiet and able to keep an almost continuous connection to the rise and fall of my breath. My body was cooperating as well, with only minor discomforts in the lower back and neck. In subsequent days, however, various physical symptoms intensified dramatically, beyond anything I had ever experienced before.

As the symptoms' intensity grew, mild anxiety gave way to a deeper part of my mind, the inner self-critic: *You're losing it—stop thinking! Stay calm, keep breathing. Come on, rally, think of something!* This inner voice looped almost continuously, interrupted only by the strike of the gong to end each session.

By day four, the pain in my lower back and now my right hip was feeling like molten, subterranean lava, slowly expanding, lifting up, forcing cracks to appear in the crust of my confidence. By the last afternoon session that day, I was feeling overwhelmed and utterly defeated. In the Q&A session that evening, I asked, "How do I escape the intense pain I'm feeling when it becomes unbearable?"

The teacher's reply: "You won't know until you go beyond what you know. Just keep going."

For the next three days of meditation, I frequently reminded myself of the opening night talk of pain as temporary in nature. It helped, a little. I was able to observe how the intensity of sensations fluctuated—sometimes increasing, sometimes decreasing, though always there to some degree. I kept telling myself, *Everything I'm experiencing will pass.* And when that wasn't enough, *No one's ever gone to the emergency room from a sitting injury!* In truth, my hopeful mind was in some denial, ignoring the fact that the periods of pain overall were increasing, even continuing during our breaks.

During the last morning session on day six, I settled into a seated crossed-leg position, and almost immediately, my right leg fell asleep. My worst fears surfaced: *Was something more serious happening?* This was followed by a cascade of other thoughts and emotions spiraling toward feelings of desperation. Unknown to me, a healing crisis/ opportunity was coming my way.

On a subconscious level, the psychological reactions to physical pain were generating a host of physiological reactions that exacerbated what I was already feeling, creating a vicious circle of intensifying pain. And before I knew it, pain had completely overwhelmed any ability to respond. A "near-death" panic was approaching: the radiating pain from my right hip was getting lost in the numbness of the leg and streaming agony up my spine; the entire musculature of my back was now gripped in full lock-down, with even the slightest movement causing nerve-searing torment. There was no escape. This would be the longest ninety minutes of my life, taking me far above any threshold of pain I'd known and deep into despair.

When I left the hall after the session, I felt like a mummy, walk-ing slowly, wrapped in the slag of my pain, head and spirit bowed, watching each of my steps forward touching the earth ahead of me but unable to feel the ground. As everyone else left the hall and turned toward lunch, I went straight into the forest, seeking the solitude I needed for the breakdown I knew was coming.

When I reached the farthest edge of the compound, out of earshot of others, I fell to my knees, screaming to a God I didn't know and had never humbled myself before: *Help me! Please! Help me!*

Silence . . . nothing. I was alone and now stripped of any self-dignity or self-worth, exhausted and humbled by sheer pain. Eventually, I stood up and walked back to my tent to lie down and rest or to sleep—it was against the rules, but following the rules at that point was useless. I was done.


## GRAVITY'S DOMAIN

The Indian *khaat* (cot) that was my bed was uncomfortably short for my body, and as I lay down on my back, my arms and legs intuitively stretched straight off the ends. I had not done yoga for nearly a week, and extending my body fully reclined, I felt like I was levitating, freed from the straightjacket of self-imposed stillness five days of sitting had created. To accommodate my large body on the small bed, I grabbed my elbows, forearms touching, and placed my arms on the bed above my head. I made a similar shape with my legs bent, shins together, feet even with my knees. The pain in my back and right hip were now only imprints, like neurological shadows of what I had felt in the hall, and with each cycle of breath, the feeling of gravity's embrace penetrated deeper—my bones, tissues, and internal organs were finally at rest.

As I lay there, wide awake, I began to feel tingling in my hands and feet. It was nothing like the pins and needles from awakening numbness after long sessions of sitting. This was different and unusually pleasant, like a warm buzz. And it wasn't static. It was slowly expanding, flowing out from my hands into my elbows and forearms, from my feet into my knees and shins. I sensed that the contact of each hand on the opposite elbow was closing an open circuit between the hands, with the forearms acting as a wire between two poles, allowing bio-electricity to flow. A similar experience was happening between my feet, connected to the opposite knees, with the shins acting as the wire.

My attention was fully absorbed in watching this unfold, and there was a bizarre sense of detachment between what my mind was witnessing and what my body was experiencing. The outer (physical) shell of my body was absolutely still, but inside was like an intracellular jamboree. I was fascinated by these alien sensations. What had initially been subtle sensation was now slowly increasing, creating a more heightened—and pleasurable—sensation that felt like warm bread dough rising, confined to the lower parts of my arms and legs.

As the sensation increased, a childlike curiosity was now fully aroused. How far would the dough rise? As the lower limbs filled, it began to ooze out of the elbows into the upper arms, and the same thing was happening out of the knees into the thighs. These two streams of inner flow slowly approached the torso from opposite ends, until the arm flow began spilling over into the shoulders and the leg flow began spilling over into the pelvis.

As the upper thoracic cavity and lower pelvic basin filled, the thought of this sensation occupying my torso to the brim stirred a distant memory of a traumatic event twelve years earlier, when I was trapped underwater, stuck in a submerged boat. This quickly interrupted the inner calm of the moment: I had a visceral impulse to escape. Panicking, I attempted to sit up on the bed, but both sets of limbs were unresponsive. Repeatedly, I tried to uncross my arms and legs, lift my head, roll to the side, but nothing happened.

As the streams of flow continued to fill my torso, my terror was real: something I felt I wasn't ready for was lurking if the two streams were to meet. With one final effort, I lunged with just enough momentum to hurl myself over the edge of the cot, freefalling to the floor twelve inches below.

I was contemplating what to do next when one of the teacher assistants walked into the tent and politely asked me what I was doing. Having no words to describe it, I mumbled that my arms and legs had fallen "asleep," and that when I attempted to get up, I fell. He helped me back up onto the bed, and after a few minutes, I regained use of my limbs. Then he asked me to come back to the hall, and to my own surprise, I said, "Sure."

To this day I can find no logical explanation for what happened next: back on my cushion, sitting cross-legged, I was free of all pain in my back and hip. At first I suspected the effects of a self-administered bio-drip of adrenaline from my terror in the tent, but this feeling continued for four more days—the physical body pain free; the mental body anxiety free, fully present, no sense of time, place, or personality, witnessing the rise and fall of my breath, the rise and fall of my thoughts, and the rise and fall of sensations.

Meditating for ten hours a day and feeling no limitations should have been a euphoric, high-five type of feeling. But strangely, there was no sense of accomplishment. I felt nothing but equanimity and gratitude. Only later did I realize the *up* side of those painful experiences on that fateful morning. Though the last session of meditation had taken me into the darkest shadows of the negativity I harbored unconsciously (*samskaras*), a few insights born out of the new perspective showed up.

While I was frozen in pain (an involuntary stillness), the urge to make physical adjustments to relieve the intensity of sensation was completely gone; I had no choice but to remain still and make space for everything that came to me. Psychologically, every thought and emotion that showed up was quickly replaced with the next as they continuously replayed the drama of it all in my mind, a reminder of the impermanence of feelings and attitudes. The sound of the gong ending the session brought an immediate and noticeable drop in the magnitude of what I was feeling—a response like Pavlov's dogs—even before I was able to move, which was also a reminder of the inseparable nature of the body and mind.

As I got up and started to move, I was sore but felt nothing acutely painful. What had felt so pathological while meditating was so transient after; and mentally, the depression I had experienced that afternoon—one of complete emptiness and, in many ways, a death of who I thought myself to be—was replaced with gratitude, peace, and a better sense of me beyond the "I."

On the last day of the program, my meditations were physically painful again, though not nearly as intense. Different this time was the lack of mental disturbance from what I was feeling—I was calm, not concerned about the physical sensations that arose; my mind was aware from a detached place of witnessing. It was similar to observing the rising of bread dough that day on the cot, without any trigger or programmed response from the subconscious part of my brain.

I saw that my mind was not an enemy to conquer. Through the voice inside that was speaking to me, a new awareness was present: The mind is a powerful tool. Its ability to self-reflect allows an impartial witnessing of behavior, whether conscious or unconscious, and the decisions about how to perceive, evaluate, or react are totally a matter of choice, just as Goenka had told us on the first night. (For more, see figure 3 on page 114.)

I also came to see that the state of deep emptiness and depression I had felt mid-retreat was nearly identical to the emptiness I was feeling now, except moving forward, there was a simultaneous sense of fullness as well—and no fear. There was an unmistakable connection between these two states of being—the former, complete emptiness with no awareness of anything except the heaviness of despair; the latter, complete emptiness with a simultaneous awareness of fullness, an interconnectedness with all things and an incredible lightness of being in body, mind, and spirit.

Though meditation and *hatha* yoga are often perceived as exclusive of one another, through this extraordinary experience, they came together for me, awakening the visceral and inseparable nature that mind and body form. Both practices open us to the latent energetic connection we have with all things.

Our ability to know things in a way that leaps over "normal" cognition and perception and just shows up as a sudden intuition . . . is an altogether logical, natural, and predictable human skill. [Our] sixth sense is simply standard-issue equipment, along with our eyes, ears, tongues, noses, and skin. It is only as magical and as ordinary as they are—which is plenty magical enough—but no more and no less.

**Belleruth Naparstek**

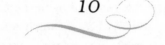

## 10

# *Our Hidden Senses— Intuition and Humor*

Now let's get back to our discussion of the senses, but this time with a different spin. Beyond the commonly understood five senses, there are two additional senses that remain mysteriously hidden from most serious scientific inquiry: the "sixth sense," or intuition, and what I refer to as the "seventh sense," our sense of humor. The former is the by-product of surrender and grace, both of which can exert influence instantaneously, with no measurable evidence, through space or time. The seventh sense is the psychological seed for levity, the psychic-emotional override that establishes balance between the heart and the brain.

## OUR SIXTH SENSE—INTUITION

Intuition and creativity have been part of my life for as long as I can remember, although only as an adult have I consciously felt their effects and noticed their accuracy. As a child, intuition took the form of either a preconception that something was going to happen or inwardly seeing something clearly and then going about making it happen. In both cases, when what I saw came to pass, it reinforced my belief in it. When it didn't work out, I felt the natural disappointment that comes when desires are left unmet.

As an adult, after years of witnessing my intuitive notions failing to happen or happening but not in the way my intuition predicted, my disappointment is now short-lived. I know that, typically, the form of universal intelligence that seems to fill the intuitive capacity of my being may have something different in store for me, above and beyond what my limited intuition has perceived, and it only requires a little more time to be realized.

Yoga, like art, is rarely discovered using the limited capacities of the individual mind alone, and it is most definitely not a linear process. It often requires turning inward, away from the physical senses and reliance on the brain's logical, analytical, detail-oriented left hemisphere. It means turning toward a vaster, deeper kind of wisdom found in the brain's nonverbal, nonlocal, artistic, "big picture"–oriented right hemisphere, as well as in the heart center, which is often referred to as the "seat of the soul" and which naturally links us to the world and the community of like-minded souls around us.

Belleruth Naparstek, whom we met in the last chapter, writes:

> Mostly, heartful practice is about keeping the heart open
> to the world around us—to people, places, ourselves, and
> the divine. It means coming from a place of empathic
> attunement. It's about seeing the connections, the
> interlocking webs of energy among people and things, and
> residing as much as possible in that place of no separation.[63]

Like Father Charlie's description of self-evident truth—a knowing that is a birthright for all of us—Naparstek writes that "it's about 'lovingness' rather than just love," that at the heart center level we can directly experience the complex ideas of theoretical physics, the interpenetrating energy fields that we are, where each vibration contains "everything in the universe, each subatomic bit of us a hologram of all that is. This is why we can experience instantaneous, direct knowing."[64]

Our ability in yoga to access the power found by surrendering into gravity and receiving the grace of intuitive response requires a vigilant awareness, an openness to the guidance that appears instantaneously with the act of releasing our often subconscious psychological grip. Naparstek writes that accessing intuition involves surrender, or "aware passivity," and she emphasizes that receptivity is required if we are to make ourselves a conduit through which intuition and all creative energies can flow.[65] This way of describing how to open to the flow of intuition is the same language to use when opening up to the flow of sensation—and to the intuitive wisdom that comes with it—in a yoga pose, with the understanding that each pose has an inherent structure that requires us to *move at will* in order to maintain the structural integrity of the pose and to prevent anatomical collapse.[66]

Shifting from active *doing* to receptive *presence*—with our perceptions turned inward, away from the outside world—is a key ingredient in developing our intuition, especially in the depths of a yoga pose or a flowing sequence of poses where attention toward balance, strength, and flexibility are required interchangeably and moment to moment, simultaneously. Turning our perceptions inward is an important component of receiving intuitive information. When we can do this, we may pass through our own interior into a vast field of higher intelligence or insight that reveals impressions or ideas on our inner "screen" of awareness. Naparstek describes four critical elements that are involved in making this shift in awareness. (The first two are my shorthand, and the last two are her words.)

- Receptive mind

- Inward focus

- "Alert attention to the subtlest and most fleeting inner impressions"

- "Acceptance of those impressions as is, without accessing, interpreting, embellishing, or noodling with them in any way"[67]

Naparstek goes on to say that "opening to [intuition] involves the paradoxical requirement of actively clearing the mind so that we can passively wait to receive information."[68] This is why passive imagination plays an important role in where we "travel," physically and psychologically, in the practice of *hatha* yoga. If we can't feel a part of our body that is psychologically stagnant, we often lack physical connection to it as well, usually due to stiffness or numbness. In that case it's helpful to visualize that part of ourselves fully involved with whatever our present level of activity is in the pose, even if that means simply following the subtle sensations that breathing creates in that area and feeling that influence by envisioning expanding, softening, or flowing, for example. With consistent practice, this creates a spark of info-energy that forges new neural pathways that grow in the direction of our mental attention or images. (In chapter 14, you will learn how to explore this on your own.)

As my relationship with Shandor deepened and the time we spent practicing privately together increased, he would, from time to time, ask me just to watch. On those days, as I have mentioned before, I learned only from the energetic exchanges that took place in the watching, something Naparstek refers to as "direct induction,"[69] with that energetic experience of the observed extending into biochemical and brain wave activity of the observer.

My practice took *quantum* leaps through our physical immediacy not only while practicing together but also on the days I observed him practice. I was experiencing what quantum science is proving—this kind of spontaneous insight is exactly what happens when the vibrations of the energy wave of our own particles come into proximity with another person's energy waves. If we are open to the other's vibration, an inevitable exchange takes place.

Most of us tend to think that our physical boundary is the outermost layer of our skin; but when we add the perspective of our energetic reality, that "border of self" gets a little fuzzy. Then, when we include the psychological boundary that our ego sets for who we are, it quickly becomes obvious that our boundaries are permeable and malleable. This is especially true when we experience the emotional states of altruism and love. In those states, we can find ourselves behaving in ways that seem to contradict our own self-defining best interests and that defy logic, until we see the possibilities that open to us when we expand our sense of self—physically, emotionally, and energetically—to include others.

## HEART-BRAIN ENTRAINMENT AND INTUITION

The HeartMath Institute in Boulder Creek, California, has studied a variation of this energetic communication between the brain and the heart, developing meditation techniques that entrain the energy patterns of the two organs. The institute's founder, Doc Lew Childre, writes that this kind of meditation "builds a standing wave of coherence between your heart, brain and body . . . uniting spirit, emotions and mind. The resulting intuitive awareness further penetrates into the domain which exists beyond time and space. In this state of internal coherence and 'amplified peace,' blocks of intuitive information can come to you in seconds."[70] This entrainment occurs when frequencies lock among heart rhythms, respiration, pulse transit time (a measure of blood pressure), and brain waves. According to HeartMath research director Rollin McCarthy, this synchronization causes brain wave patterns to slow down to frequencies around 0.1 hertz and below. It is at these very low frequencies that great power resides for healing, perceptual shifts, experience reprocessing, and intuiting.[71]

HeartMath meditations use guided imagery, combining both memories and bodily sensations. Subjects are first asked to envision breathing through their hearts, a form of kinesthetic imagery that keeps their focus physically heart centered. Then they mentally reconnect with a memory that generates loving feelings, an interim step to directly accessing those feelings. Similarly in yoga, when you create mental images (energetic presence) of inactive or subconscious parts of yourself being touched with the cool, subtle expansion of your inhaling breath or of warm softness (physically) or empathy (psychologically) with your exhaling breath, the awareness of slow, soft breathing itself can create physical and neurological shifts. This, in turn, can open the door to bursts of intuitive insight that you would otherwise miss and that will further inform your practice.

What is this intelligent energy that streams in when we dissolve our boundaries in these ways? Naparstek sees "a sea of seamless, vibrating energy, alive and pulsing with omniscient, nonlocal, and infinite intelligence."[72] She concludes that "this description of an infinite sea of intelligent energy with properties of ubiquity, infinity, and omniscience sounds an awful lot like anybody's basic description of God."[73]

Astounding as it is, this is the realization we arrive at with the practice of yoga and awareness of the *koshas* of consciousness in our body. Each step deeper into these subtle body layers of ourselves gives us a progressively more refined understanding of self, until we reach the deep still point of equanimity—the ultimate awareness of our spirit/bliss field (*anandamaya kosha*), the permeating vibration of love. This energy of love is what Father Charlie referred to as "gravity" and described as "the energy of bonding"—the universal force that brings and holds us together. Could the forces of love and gravity be one and the same, energetically speaking?

Intuition arrives in many forms and through a variety of means. In many ways, its info-energy is alive and, as such, cannot be predicted. It is a mystery that escapes logic yet produces incredible insight. And it seems to appear only when we are ready to receive it, open to the idea of it, and sensitive to its subtleties.

Luckily, such was my state when I chanced across a biography of Itzhak Bentov, mentioned earlier in the book. I had conjectured in drafting this section that the scientists of the future would also be practitioners of spiritual traditions such as yoga and meditation and that these practices would help them report on the science of spiritual practices firsthand. I discovered that Bentov was an accomplished meditator; was fascinated with the links among science, the workings of our brain, the mind, and spirituality; and was an early exponent of consciousness studies.[74] So it felt appropriate to let him wrap up this discussion of intuition with one of his observations about yoga:

> To function on this level [of love] is the goal of all yoga training. The word "yoga" means union, by which is meant union with the absolute. An accomplished yogi is able to function on all levels of creation; to describe events in the

past and future; and, because the energy-exchange curve is very high on this level, he is able to influence Nature in a positive way. Eventually, he becomes a factor stimulating evolution of mankind and of the planet. . . . [The yogi] praises the spiritual level of consciousness and the rewards of those who achieve it. But this does not mean that the universe is spiritual. The universe just *is*. . . . What we call spiritual development is the key to achieving a subjective and objective understanding of the universe.[75]

## OUR SEVENTH SENSE: HUMOR

To me, don't take yourself too seriously is the same thing as Buddha recommending non-attachment. When we're in a posture of seriousness, we're very attached to the belief, the practice that we're taking seriously. Learning to replace seriousness with some playfulness is a great practice of non-attachment.

**J. P. Sears**

As a young teacher of Iyengar yoga, a style that is very precise and "serious," I couldn't have imagined that thirty years later, humor and lightheartedness, or what I refer to as *levity*, would be a fundamental theme of my teaching. Happily, since those early days, scientists have gathered evidence for why levity is beneficial in yoga and in so many other areas of life. In this way, I suppose, the evolutionary gift of laughter, accorded uniquely to the human species, has become a serious matter. Laughter, it turns out, contributes to brain-heart coherence and to the release of bioactive neuropeptides, which decrease stress hormones while increasing immune cells and antibodies that fight infection and inflammation. And that's just the start of the good news.

Importantly for me, the scientific investigation into humor has given my "inner dork-ness" permission to reveal itself and soften the way-too-serious-ness that had infected my yoga practice and teaching from the start. Teaching and learning are both a lot more fun (and productive) when you lighten up.

Let's return for a moment to Paul Pearsall. In *The Heart's Code*, he describes an episode of uncontrollable laughter he shared with a nurse tending to him when he was undergoing a routine treatment for stage 4 lymphoma, a deadly form of cancer of the lymph system. Amid such dire circumstances, Pearsall was gifted the spontaneous warmth and joy of shared good humor, and for days after, he felt its positive effects. He writes, "As my nurse indicated by saying our laughter was 'killing her' as she lost all sense of self-control, humor, much like loving and sensual connection . . . is a form of 'selfless resonance' of a heart-to-heart subtle [body] energy connection."[76] In the moment of heart connection shared through loss of self-control, Pearsall experienced a "jocular epiphany"—an event of cardio-coherence where "the brain's illusion of its ultimate control [and arrogance] over our destiny is exposed."[77]

Intense humor can act as a window, beyond the ego-mind's limited view, into the quantum field, where, as author James Gleick observes, "Just beneath the apparent order of the universe, there is chaos and at the same time, within that chaos, there is an order we are still far from understanding."[78] Pearsall adds to this idea:

> Cardio-energetics suggests that our heart is sensitive to the dynamic hidden order beneath the chaos and, when it finds it, it often makes us laugh until we cry at our recognition of our brain's foolish pride in its illusion of mastery of destiny. Through its hard, tear-inducing laughter, the heart tells us that, for at least a few moments, our "self" as perceived by the brain has escaped the stress of life and temporarily "died" laughing and gone to quantum heaven.[79]

Many cultures around the world have recognized the tension between the chaos of living and the rational plans our brain uses to avoid life's turmoil and the heart's capacities to make peace with that tension.

Pearsall writes of the mythical demigod Maui, whom native Hawaiians called "the Trickster," a figure who constantly makes mischief tricking others. Pearsall notes how widespread the trickster is in the mythology of indigenous cultures:

> We need the trickster's little jokes on us to remind us to pay more attention to the gift of being alive. . . . He teaches us about who we are and what we can and can never be, even if his lessons are often clumsy and disturbing to our plans and image of who our brain thinks we are. Our brain would like to keep the trickster out of our life, but our heart knows well how to play, learn, and laugh with the trickster.[80]

Integrating regular doses of humor into our life, our practice, and our yoga is one of the easiest and most efficient ways to establish beneficial changes in the neurochemistry of our brain and bring about consistent heart-brain coherence, especially if we are experiencing a life-threatening disease. Author Norman Cousins, who healed himself from several such illnesses, in part using humor, writes, "Of all the gifts bestowed by nature on human beings, hardy laughter must be close to the top."[81]

We've all heard the adage "laughter is the best medicine." Laughter truly is one of the most underrated tools in our healing repertoire—free, readily available, with no unwanted side effects, and now substantiated by a growing body of research. According to Pearsall, one study has shown that twenty seconds of guffawing gives the heart the same beneficial workout as three minutes of hard rowing; other studies have indicated that even people hearing laughter experience benefits, too.[82]

As a teacher, I find the use of humor, like the act of teaching itself, a very intuitive exercise, involving pauses that appear in the stream of thoughts or spoken words used to communicate a concept or idea, pauses that allow other info-energy to flow. The process opens up opportunities to respond in the moment; to observe what is present in the class; to receive energetic signals from the students' presence, moods, energies, comments, and questions; and to follow what comes naturally in response.

As my abilities to find humor have developed, I have seen that, like intuition, humor is never 100 percent "on point," especially when it comes to timing. So when a "serious" attempt at intuitive humor falls flat, I try to stay in the moment and respond to the students' sometimes confused silence in a fully present way. I often wait until the silence is deafening and then say something like, "Yes, in case you didn't realize, that was an attempt at humor." I may go on to explain that good humor requires a sophisticated audience that is familiar with the fine arts of nuance and subtlety, and that when my humor is beyond my audience's abilities, I usually resort to bad humor! This is always good for a short burst of nervous laughter, the kind of laughter we habitually resort to when someone we care about tells a bad joke. Surprisingly, even "bad" humor (think "dad jokes") can initiate the necessary energetic shift and has the potential to produce effects on our nervous system similar to "good" humor.

Integrating humor or lightheartedness into your practice when you're by yourself is a different matter, of course. It's not so much about telling jokes to yourself; rather, it has more to do with not taking yourself too seriously. Although yoga practice often requires strong resolve, not being intensely serious about it makes time spent practicing more enjoyable. But how can you do that?

Start by taking your time. Build pauses into your practice—when it comes to levity, there's no rush. Then use your imaginative powers of visualization. Here are some suggestions:

- To create more easeful breathing, you can "smell the roses" by imagining a fragrant rose blossom, or any aromatic flower of your choice, under your nostrils.

- To create more fluid movement, imagine the marrow inside your bones or the connective tissue within and around your muscles as being soft.

- To more fully connect to the ground and relaxation, picture the major bones and internal organs in your body heavy and deeply at rest.

- For more lightness of being, feel the inner spaciousness of your joints or hollow organs when exhaling slowly.

Releasing the "serious muscle" in our minds means we can relax our need to be right or follow the "rules" perfectly. When we introduce these types of pauses in our practice, we open ourselves to new possibilities, new ways to see what we are feeling, and new ways to interpret and influence what we are feeling. And maybe the best thing to introduce, or reintroduce, into your practice is to be okay with the mystery of it, to be curious about exploring and seeing for yourself, beyond any rules you may have learned about "correctness" or style.

# PART 4

## Subtle Body Anatomy

What exactly is the subtle body in yoga? What are its main components, and where are they located? How can we work with subtle body anatomy as yoga practitioners? This is the focus of part 4. In this next chapter, we'll start with the subtle body system that may be most familiar to you: the *chakras*. But before we get there, let's take a step back—or maybe a step up—to look at what makes up a human being.

### LESSONS FROM VIPASSANA

During the first-night introduction of the Vipassana meditation retreat (for more, see chapter 9), we watched a video of Goenka speaking. The topic of his talk? Nothing less than the very nature of who we are.

He spoke in great detail about how our physical body appears solid and how what we think and feel seem indisputable, but the reality is entirely different. He said that our true nature is a composite of five processes, one physical and the other four mental (see figure 3 on next page).

Science has now shown us that the physical matter of our bodies—anything physical, in fact—is actually a combination of subatomic particles and empty space. In addition, the life span of these subatomic particles is less than a trillionth of a second; all are repeatedly being born, dying, and being reborn. Goenka shared that the Buddha knew this twenty-five hundred years ago:

The entire material universe was comprised of particles, called *kalapas* [in Pali], or "indivisible units." These units exhibit in endless variation the basic qualities of matter: mass, cohesion, temperature, and movement. They combine to form structures which seem to have some permanence. But actually these are all composed of minuscule *kalapas* which are in a state of continuously arising and passing away.[83]

As a pragmatist, Goenka strove for simple explanations. He shared how the Buddha examined his own mental processes through meditation, discovering in broad, simple terms four steps we use to integrate information received through our five senses of sight, sound, smell, taste, and touch. The first step is *consciousness*, which

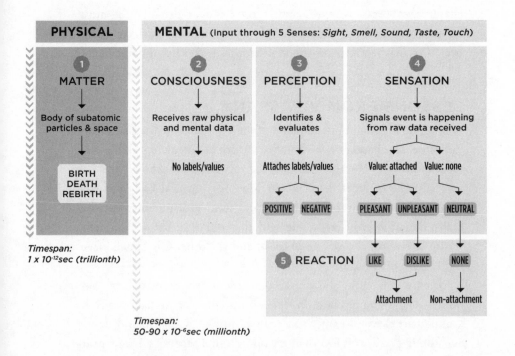

**FIGURE 3** The five processes of human being

the Buddha defined as the part of our mind that registers the occurrence of any phenomenon—the receipt of any input, physical or mental; it does so without assigning labels or value judgments. The second step is *perception*, or the act of recognition, which identifies whatever has been noted by consciousness and proceeds to distinguish it with a label and then evaluate it as either positive or negative. The next step in mental processing is *sensation*, which is the signal the body uses to alert the mind that something is happening. As long as the signal is not evaluated, the sensation remains neutral. However, once a value is attached to the input, the sensation becomes pleasant or unpleasant. Pleasant sensations create desire to prolong or intensify the experience, while unpleasant sensations (pain) create the desire to stop it or avoid it.

Once the value is established, the last mental process is *reaction*: if the sensation is pleasant, the mind reacts with a like; if the sensation is unpleasant, the mind reacts with a dislike; and if the sensation is neutral, there is no reaction. (This will be a useful perspective to have when you get to the concept of *samskaras* in the next chapter.)

For the unexamined mind, mental reactions are experienced as if they are reality, in a similar way to our experience when encountering a physical part of our body we can touch that feels real. What Goenka conveyed to me that first night was that the impermanence of sensations is no different from the impermanence of thought, and the time span for each of these occurrences is so short that we cannot perceive that they are constantly reoccurring. Despite appearances, the true reality of ourselves is an unbroken progression of closely connected events that give the appearance of continuity, solidity, and identity. In other words, who we *think* we are is not really who we are.

Goenka closed his talk that night with the Buddha's realization that our true reality, physically and mentally, is not a finished, unchanging *being* but an unfinished and continuous process of *becoming*, flowing from moment to moment.

With the practice of yoga and meditation, we come to realize that the external reality is a reality, but only a superficial one. At a deeper level, the reality is that the entire universe, animate and inanimate, is in a constant state of becoming—of arising and passing away.

Each of us is, in fact, a stream of constantly changing subatomic particles, along with the processes of consciousness, perception, sensation, and reaction, which are also changing at a speed that blurs this reality, hidden below the appearances of permanence.

~

This is our fundamental nature as the human yoga practitioners we all are. It is helpful to keep this construct in mind as we learn to activate the subtle body in our practice.

Chakra theory goes to the deepest sources of all dynamic processes in man, down to the deepest cosmic functions, to which we are all undeniably bound. There are many effects resulting from the activity of the [central nervous system] and the glands which will forever remain a mystery if we ignore the much subtler aspects of [the] chakras.

**Hans Ulrich Rieker**

## 11

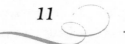

# Subtle Body "Seats of Energy Consciousness" — the Chakras

The *chakra* system has ancient origins. Those who first came to understand how it functions did so thousands of years before modern science began to recognize the nonmechanistic view of the body's intricate bio-electrochemical energy system and how it works synchronistically with our brain, organs, and glands to maintain health and equilibrium (homeostasis). Today, the more science discovers, the more it confirms how yoga affects the health of our bodies and, curiously, how science and yoga have more interconnection than had been imagined. There are complexities and mysteries within both yoga and science that often defy logical explanation. Instead, intuition and the perception of self-evident truths are required to approach an understanding.

As I learned more about *chakras*—the seats of energy consciousness in our subtle body—I struggled to make sense of how I could apply that knowledge while practicing on my mat or going about my life. For me, the concepts were vague, and the terminology and philosophy of different lineages of yoga and *Ayurveda* were often contrary. I ran across different views of the composition, location, number, and function of the *chakras*. There were various opinions and beliefs about how to open them: which vocal or subvocal sounds to chant, which objects or colors to visualize, which exercises to use, and whether the mystical experience of *kundalini*—thought of as a dormant spiritual energy visualized as a coiled snake asleep at the base of the spine—was to be either intentionally sought after or avoided as an unnecessary distraction.

The visualizations I tried first were based on something I had read in several books that sounded cool: the idea of *chakras* as whirling vortexes of colored energy or light. Following a system that seemed to have a random consensus, I devoted several hours a week to sitting in meditation, my inner gaze focused on creating these mini-cyclones of cosmic luminosity in seven locations. It was fun to do but hard to actually feel. When that felt unproductive, I would just "wing it" a bit, which didn't help much either.

Reading about the *chakra* system or listening to teachers speak about it gave me some clues of what to look for, but for my first few years of practice, it felt like nothing was "happening." My mind was frustrated trying to find agreement among all the yogis who addressed *chakras*. Eventually I gave up my esoteric search and turned my focus back toward simpler goals, such as pounding away at my chronically tight, steel-belted hamstrings; getting my hips open enough to sit comfortably in lotus position, which seemed to be an important part of meditating; and learning how to do those cool-looking, free-balancing handstands. At the time, achieving those latter poses seemed to be a particularly special skill to have as an aspiring yoga teacher, especially for pictures on workshop fliers to attract attention and validate that I was a qualified teacher: "Hey, look at that. This guy must know his stuff!" I thought that maybe once my body had opened enough through *asana*, I would finally understand *chakras*, and they would "automatically" awaken.

Years later, having made varying degrees of progress in those simple goals, I came to notice areas of accumulated emotional residue in the form of chronic tension in my body that the style of yoga I was practicing was not adequately addressing—patterns of stress that would return within a day or two if I missed my daily practice, or areas that were so blocked I felt complete physical numbness there, even with consistent practice. The areas that held the most resistance to feeling were my pelvic floor, diaphragm, and throat. I'd had physical sports injuries in those areas, too (tailbone, lower back, and neck), and I began to see that the two might be related. Perhaps my physical injuries had caused a level of psychological anxiety that would not allow me to fully relax there. Or maybe some of the psychological traumas and stresses of ordinary life that I'd experienced hadn't been fully cleared from my sympathetic nervous system and had burrowed their way into the connective tissues there, maybe even contributing to the physical weakness at the root of those injuries. In those days, I could find no doctors who were open to that kind of conversation, but my yoga studies were revealing to me that such connections were more than likely.

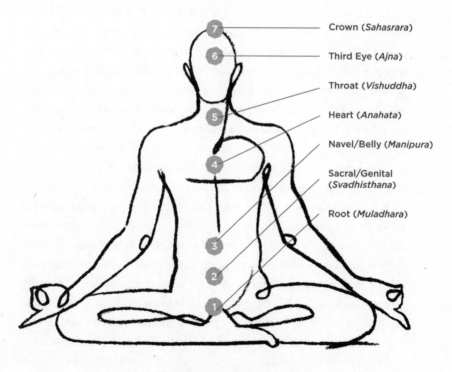

Crown (*Sahasrara*)

Third Eye (*Ajna*)

Throat (*Vishuddha*)

Heart (*Anahata*)

Navel/Belly (*Manipura*)

Sacral/Genital (*Svadhisthana*)

Root (*Muladhara*)

**FIGURE 4**  *Chakras*

I could see those connections, but I was still unclear how to go about unwinding the specific subconscious stresses in those particular areas in any sustainable way. I was becoming aware that even after practice and a great sense of calm in my trouble spots, I had a sense that I was missing the root of residual subconscious tension, as though I were feebly attempting to pull the weeds in my garden of trouble spots, and that was why my "stuff" returned when I wasn't practicing. I wondered: How could my yoga practice help me reset the baseline of the relaxation response in my nervous system lower than what I had become accustomed to? How could it affect change in the areas I couldn't feel at all?

Then the day came when I realized that although it was important to use the power of my creative mind when practicing, it wasn't important in the way I would have thought. I had to first let go of expectations, intentions, and goals, while still hanging on to my commitment to practice, and simply remain curious about what showed up.

At the start of this new approach, I found it remarkable that the *chakras* were located in such close proximity to the major glands and organs of the body's endocrine system and the major nerve plexuses. Was that a mere coincidence? Until that point, I hadn't made a strong connection between the physical work of stretching and strengthening my muscles and the mental work of stretching and strengthening my mind. It took an act of surrender in the "control center" of my brain to realize that my *body* had a mind (or minds) of its own and that my organs and glands played much bigger roles in consciousness than Western science's love of the omnipresent mind in the brain could explain.

It is now so obvious to me that, like yoga itself, the *chakras* are very personal and unique to the individual. To appreciate what exactly they are and how they work within you involves creating an image of them in your mind—including both visuals and sounds—and applying your unique understanding of them. When that is your practice, eventually your relationship with your *chakras* will awaken a feeling sense of non-muscular, subtle body movement within. If this produces a truth for you that your life benefits from, then the *chakras* will become *real* to you.

In his studies of Sanskrit, tantric yoga, and classical Indian philosophy, teacher and scholar Christopher Wallis explains:

The *chakras* aren't like organs in the physical body; they aren't fixed facts that we can study like doctors study neural ganglia (with which the *chakras* were confused in the nineteenth century). The energy body (*suksma sarira*) is an extraordinarily fluid reality, as we should expect of anything nonphysical and supersensuous. The energy body can present, experientially speaking, with any number of energy centers, depending on the person and the yogic practice they're performing.[84]

Wallis's research confirmed for me that much of what is taught about *chakras* by Western *hatha* yoga teachers involves practices that have been co-opted from references to old traditional texts, overlaid with modern Western psychological states innovated by Carl Jung in the 1930s, with very little relevance to the culturally specific context from which the original practices were born. In fact, many Western students have had, and continue to have, powerful experiences doing practices that have no solid basis in recognized traditions. So I appreciate Dr. Wallis's advice to Western yoga teachers:

> When it comes to the chakras, don't claim you know. Tell your yoga students that every book on the chakras presents only one possible model. Nothing written in English is really authoritative for practitioners of yoga. So why not hold more gently the beliefs you've acquired about yoga, even while you keep learning? Let's admit we really don't understand these ancient yoga practices yet; and instead of seeking to be an authority on some oversimplified version of them, you can invite yourself and your students to look more clearly, more honestly, more carefully, and more non-judgmentally at their own inner experience.[85]

This was the approach I stumbled onto: to step back from what I thought I knew about *chakras* and be more present and intimate with my own inner experiences of these mystical, esoteric landmarks in the body.

I have to say, though, that my initial, limited experiences were mostly unpleasant. With more focused attention in the three regions I mentioned, I began to see that the continuous subconscious grip that held even the smallest amount of emotional tension or subtle muscular contraction was a literal waste of energy. The unnecessary muscular effort it took to hold on to the psycho-physical contractions was slowly leaking my life-force energy. And I could feel that the effects of continuous subtle body contraction would inevitably have a physical effect on the proper functioning of associated endocrine glands, nerve synapses, and organs in those areas, making them work harder to function normally. It was like you'd expect the lungs to feel when you're breathing deeply in a straitjacket or what your voice might sound like if you were singing with your mouth covered by a pillow.

Recognizing how contraction in these areas could sap my energy, I stepped back from the practice of *bandhas*, translated as "locks" or "binds." These practices of deliberate contraction in the body were meant to intensify life-force energy, but was there any irony there? Could it be that the zeal with which I practiced *bandhas* was partly responsible for my inability to feel full release in those areas? I was about to put all my practice cards on the table. Could I discover other possibilities for my practice that held keys to the remaining centers of consciousness in my body? That was my hope.

The practice of yoga is directed at awakening the divine energy within every human being. Asanas and Pranayama uncoil and alert the chakras. In the process the nadis are activated. This causes the chakras to vibrate and generate energy, which is then circulated all over the body through the nadis. The emotions rooted in the chakras are transformed as divine energies awakened and circulated.

B. K. S. Iyengar

# UP FROM THE MUCK: A BLOSSOM

The well-known symbol representing the *chakras* is the lotus blossom. The lotus flower plant naturally grows in swampy, stagnant water, usually under dark, murky conditions, its roots embedded in rotting pond sludge. Incredibly, though, as it grows upward, it awakens into the light at the surface as a delightful flower of intense beauty and purity, tethered by a strong, flexible stem grounding it firmly into the muck of its origins.

It's no wonder this flower is such a potent symbol for many spiritual traditions around the world. In Buddhism, the lotus bud symbolizes potential. The lotus flower represents spiritual growth and enlightenment. This plant's circumstances offer a perfect metaphor for obstacles becoming gifts, for moving through the dank recesses within to find the brilliance of the inner light that abounds. As I continued to explore *chakras*, the "mucky" areas of my body I had felt limited by were starting to yield flashes of insight to go further.

In yoga philosophy, our psychic-emotional muck is known as *samskaras*. My feelings of being stuck or numb to these subconscious gifts motivated me to continue laying bare what was uncomfortable to admit—that there was still more material for my inner work to address, that there were areas that required showing up for and a deeper quality of relationship with. Dr. Wallis sees the yogic theory of *samskaras* as "one of India's most fascinating contributions to our understanding of human psychology." He says,

> When we experience aversion to a painful experience, or attachment to a pleasurable one, an impression of that experience is laid down in our psyche, which is said to be a "seed" of experience which will sprout again. . . . In other words, when we are unable to fully "show up" for any given experience, a remnant of it is deposited in our psyche—or, in Tantrik theory, in the "subtle body" which is simply the extension of the psyche. The subtle body is said to interpenetrate and underlie the physical body in the sense that it is a model for explaining how unresolved past experiences shape our relationship to the body (and its health) in the present.[86]

Without the awareness of how our *samskaras* influence and obscure our mind's abilities to clearly perceive our reality, we hamstring our growth toward a true sense of life and who we are. Though Wallis admits his descriptions may be oversimplified, he concludes,

> Everyone carries around with them a whole host of *samskaras* from this lifetime and previous lives (since the subtle body does not die with the physical one), and those impressions unconsciously shape our preferences and the assumptions we project onto the people and situations we encounter. The stronger the emotional impact of an experience, the deeper the impression that is formed, until we end up with a whole network of impressions that function as a filter to reality.[87]

## EXPERIMENTATION

After a strong practice of postures one morning followed by a long relaxation on the floor and a short session of *pranayama*, I was inspired to test an idea I'd had the night before. Recalling the experiences I had while healing my lower back and applying what I had learned from Vipassana meditation, I took a comfortable, seated, cross-legged position and began focusing first on the pelvic floor. I directed my attention to follow the slow, gentle expansion of my inhaling breath through my back and the full length of my torso, visualizing the subtle wind (*vayu*) of my breath moving through the subtle central channel associated with my spine (*sushumna nadi*, the primary conduit of the *chakra* system). I visualized it energetically filling into and through my rectum and the fullness of my subtle breath gently pressing the perineum (the gateway to the first *chakra*, *muladhara*) into the floor. On the exhaling breath, I placed my full attention into *consciously softening* deep into my pelvic floor and sphincter muscles, both urinary and anal. Then I moved my attention with the retreat of the outgoing breath, up through the back, while consciously softening the skin below my navel (gateway to the second *chakra*, *svadhisthana*), my diaphragm (gateway to the third *chakra*, *manipura*), the top of my lungs and sternum (gateway to the fourth *chakra*, *anahata*), the root of the throat and thyroid gland (gateway to the fifth *chakra, vishuddha*), and finally the nasal passages, optic muscles behind my eyes, and the frontal lobe tissues of the brain (gateway to the sixth *chakra, ajna*).

I left the crown of the head (gateway to the seventh *chakra, sahasrara*) out of the equation, for no other reason than it felt beyond my understanding of what I was drawn to do. What I did feel drawn to do was to forget about the lotus images, the colors, and the subvocal mantras I had read about for now; instead, I developed a relationship with the parts of me that were "real"—the sound of my breath and images of the organs, glands, and connective tissue proximal to the pelvic floor, the abdominal cavity, the thoracic cavity, the throat, and the "stuff" inside my head.

Then, as I did, when I used images to work with a tight muscle or an injured joint, I focused and fully embodied softening into the pelvic floor (my connection to ground) with the warm, releasing energy of exhaling.

I felt an immediate and localized sensation of "inner space." It felt like another dimension of outer space, like a celestial black hole opening within, and I funneled my attention there deeply. Inside that space, there were no images, no thoughts, just emptiness—and it felt amazing! I was feeling "space" or "nothing," a completely different experience from the lack of feeling I was used to. To try to put it into words, "bliss" or the "energy of love" come closest.

After several cycles of breathing this way, I moved my focus to the diaphragm and repeated the same process, first following the incoming breath through my back-body the full length of my torso, and on the outgoing breath, focusing my attention and conscious softening directed at the natural release of the diaphragm when exhaling. Once again, I moved my attention with the retreating breath, step by step, from the diaphragm to the top of the lungs, the root of the throat, up through the nasal passages, and back out through the nostrils. Again, I experienced localized bliss and feelings of "inner space." I repeated this process with the throat, and then with each of the remaining locations. Each time, the experience produced a level of calm and sense of abounding freedom and lightness, not only in each place of focus but also throughout. I sensed that the subtle life-force energy I felt moving was the very same energy that was being used to restrain the unmet emotions (*samskaras*) trapped in the connective tissues of my body.

This wasn't just a physical feeling. I felt that space had been cleared—a sense of lightness had appeared—in the whole of my psychological being through the unleashing of repressed emotional reaction. There was a subtle sense of unrecognizable energy released from deep within my subconscious, transformed out of past moments of unresolved emotions like greed, anger, self-interest, or fear and the reactions they created in me. Patanjali's *Yoga Sutras* mention these emotions as obstacles to the practice of yoga; I was now seeing these obstacles in a different light.

In this light, I saw that having a different relationship to our emotional triggers is possible, that they actually embody healing opportunities to *reset our mind-set*. It is possible to apprehend the guise of our *samskaras* with patience, suspending the need to judge or react, and reframe the way we respond—not from the emotional dregs of the past embedded into the subconscious playback device in the brain, but from the present-moment expression of what is true now from a state of equanimity of conscious thought. This is the place where we can begin a process of dissolving and moving beyond similar confrontations in the future.

I had learned through experimentation what Christopher Wallis maintains: when exploring the subtle body, the first order of business is to suspend judgment, because judgments are a form of resistance to reality—and resistance reinforces *samskaras*.[88] When you can do this in practice regarding *chakras*, you don't need to wrestle with competing ideas of location for this, sound for that, color for this, and try to come to a conclusion. Your inner intelligence will find its own way to the truths your subtle body holds; in cooperation with your physical body (*sthula sarira*), you will come to recognize your own ways to creatively apply yourself physically, mentally, and emotionally to find expression of *chakras* for healing in your everyday life.

In the simplest terms, *asanas*, or postures, are designed
to open the *nadis*. *Pranayama* [breathing exercises]
enables us to increase *prana* within us and direct it
as a cleansing force that eliminates impurities.

T. K. V. Desikachar

*12*

# Subtle Body "Channels" — the Nadis

As B. K. S. Iyengar's quote in the last chapter suggests, a sense of
uncoiling, physically and psychologically, in the space around and
within the *chakras* provides a window into other components of
the subtle body, starting with activation of the subtle channels or
"streams" called *nadis*. These channels allow the more refined aspects
of our vital life force to flow and circulate with less resistance, while
supporting the essential energies responsible for life, matter, mind,
and consciousness.

Refined *pranic* forces flowing though the subtle body's invisible
network of *nadis* are the means by which the subtle and the gross in
the human organism meet.[89] Of the numerous subtle channels found
in our bodies, three are of greatest significance. There is the primary
channel known as *sushumna* (Sanskrit for "gracious" or "kind"),
which runs within the full length of the spinal cord, connecting each
*chakra* from the first (*muladhara*) at the base up to and terminating
at the seventh (*sahasrara*) at the crown of the head. Then there are
two secondary channels that help regulate breathing. *Ida* (Sanskrit for

"heaven/celestial space" or "offering"), known as the moon channel and associated with feminine principles and cooling energies, connects the left side of the body with the right hemisphere of the brain. It controls our parasympathetic nervous system, supplies energy to the heart, and terminates in the left nostril. *Pingala* (Sanskrit for "Earth/material universe" or "austerity") is known as the sun channel. It is associated with masculine principles and warming energies and connects the right side of the body with the left hemisphere of the brain. It controls our sympathetic nervous system, supplies energy to the brain, and terminates in the right nostril. The interconnectedness of our nostrils with the opposite hemispheres of our brain suggests the influence *pranayama* can have on the brain's autonomic nervous system, restoring balance to sympathetic and parasympathetic functions.

*Nadis* can be stimulated by direct, physical touch at energy points (*marmas*) on the surface of the skin and by indirect, psychic-emotional "touch" through visualization (thoughts), feelings (emotions), or any form of intangible transmission of subtle energy (sensations) found within the nonphysical *chakra* system. Once engaged through conscious practices like yoga, meditation, or massage, these subtle channels carry the flow of vibrational thought-energy (*prana vayu*), which can offer support for local symptoms found around a specific point; travel to remote physiological targets such as organs and glands; or just help reset the overall well-being of the body and mind, unfolding the body's natural ability to heal. More important, the *nadis* carry information that unveils and confirms the undeniable continuity between body and mind, energy and consciousness.

Using this information while practicing yoga is not as complex as it might first appear. Though there are estimated to be 72,000 *nadis* in our body, establishing a manageable working relationship with the three better-known channels mentioned above—one primary and two secondary—is a good place to start. Patanjali's *Yoga Sutras* offer guidance on how to establish a rapport with the principles found in these channels, using conscious breathing and movement, awareness of thoughts and emotions, and a basic understanding of *chakras* and subtle body anatomy.

The three channels carry psychic-emotional energy and operate in a nonphysical realm. In this environment, our thoughts and emotions are energy—the same energy that manifests in the physical matter of our bodies. If we habitually dwell on negative thoughts and emotions, the flow of psychic-emotional energy is of a lower vibration and slows down. If this pattern is left unchecked, the energy begins to stagnate. Over time, this stagnation can have a negative effect on the physiological systems of the body that depend on healthy levels of vibration in these psychic-emotional channels. Eventually, the body will speak through the only language it knows for communicating imbalance, beginning with minor symptoms of pain. If we are unaware of or misunderstand our body's attempt to communicate, it communicates more loudly with increasing symptoms until we intervene.

If we wait too long, we have to seek outside medical help to alleviate or suppress our symptoms so that our life can get back to "normal." But if we don't understand how the thought mechanisms of our subtle body work and do not find ways to interrupt the low-vibration energy of habitual negative thoughts, the symptoms will inevitably return.

## THE MOVEMENT OF THOUGHTS AND EMOTIONS

Essentially, our thoughts are divided into two types. The first is thinking about concrete objects or things, like which clothes to wear today or what you ate for breakfast. These thoughts tend to occupy the secondary channel, *pingala*. Then there is thinking about the mind itself: thinking about your mind thinking about things, or awareness of the miracle that our minds can think or sense anything at all. These thoughts tend to occupy the secondary channel, *ida*.

As figure 5 shows, the primary (central) energetic channel, *sushumna*, is located within the main physical network of our body's bioelectrical nervous system, running centrally through the full length of our spine. Most schools of traditional and modern yoga are in general agreement about the location and function of this channel, though with various ideas about how to awaken the dormant spiritual energy that resides at the base of the spine (*kundalini*).

In contrast, there is much debate over the two secondary channels: how they function; where they are located; how they travel around, alongside, or across points along the spine; and whether they move to peripheral areas beyond the central channel of the spine. What I share here is my current state of understanding, based on personal experience and research on a variety of Indian and Western translations associated with the *Yoga Sutras*. I acknowledge that this is a work in progress, as should be anything that is alive and part of the cosmic mystery tour we are all participants in.

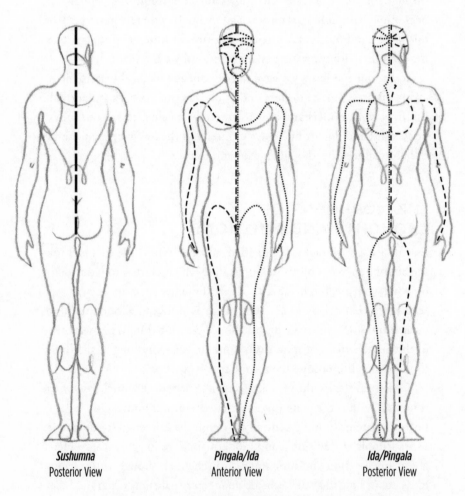

*Sushumna*
Posterior View

*Pingala/Ida*
Anterior View

*Ida/Pingala*
Posterior View

**FIGURE 5** The primary and secondary channels: *nadis*

For each of the following sutras quoted below, I list the original Sanskrit transliteration followed by an English translation to avoid confusion, as numbering systems of the sutras can differ. The translations presented here come from Michael Roach and Christie McNally's *The Essential Yoga Sutra: Ancient Wisdom for Your Yoga*.[90] These translations have a simplistic quality to them that might be unsatisfying to traditionalists, but I personally resonate with them. They speak to my own decades of thought, training, and meditation and the effects those years of practice have had on the changing landscape of my ego attachments and the deconstruction of much of the personality I used to strongly identify with.

## Insight about *Pingala Nadi* (The Masculine Channel)

*Sutra III.26: Bhuvanajnanam surye samyamat.*

> Turn the combined effort
> upon the sun,
> and you will understand
> the earth (our world).

The channel of the sun, to the right side of our central channel, carries the inner "winds" of our negative, heated thoughts and emotions—such as anger, hatred, fear, jealousy—which involve largely masculine energy (externally focused and action oriented). These create disliking and blind aversion to objects—such as things, events, and people. Understanding this concept and the awareness of the psychic-emotional residue that results helps us begin to see and ultimately control the very thoughts we have produced through misunderstanding our outer reality: the "earth—the world that we live in."[91] Our misunderstanding is the belief that the world is other and separate from who we are (that is, physical-solid reality versus energetic-quantum reality), and it occurs when we believe in the programs (or seeds) that are planted in our subconscious through misperceptions. Stilling these mental disturbances simply and effectively through the practice of *hatha* yoga and *pranayama* (breathing exercises) helps free us from the outside in; meditation and inner knowledge of our true outer world helps free us from the inside out.

## Insight about *Ida Nadi* (The Feminine Channel)

*Sutra III.27: Candre tara vyuha jnanam.*

> You will understand
> the arrangement of the stars
> if you turn this same effort
> upon the moon.

The channel of the moon, to the left side of our central channel, carries the inner "winds" of our negative, obsessive thoughts or emotions—the reactions or feelings we can't escape concerning the things, events, or people that involve largely feminine energy (introspective and emotionally oriented). These create "liking" and blind attachments to emotions—for example, the way our minds instinctively believe our perceptions of our circumstances. Understanding this concept and the awareness of the psychic-emotional residue that results helps us see and ultimately control the very thoughts we produced through misunderstanding our inner reality: the "stars—the tiny sparks of consciousness within us"[92] that we believe are real and are who we are. For example, "I am angry," instead of "I am experiencing feelings of anger." Like imbalances in the sun channel, our misunderstanding comes from the "seeds" planted within our subconscious programming. Stilling these mental disturbances simply and effectively through the practice of *hatha* yoga and *pranayama* helps free us from the outside in; meditation and inner knowledge helps free us from the inside out.

## Insight about *Sushumna Nadi* (The Main Central Channel)

*Sutra III.28: Dhruve tadgati jnanam.*

> Turn the effort
> upon the polestar,
> and you will understand
> their workings.

The central channel carries the inner "winds" of graciousness, kindness, and all the positive thoughts we share in being human, such as love, gratitude, compassion, joy, and equanimity. Its axis runs centrally in our bodies, like a polestar upon which our world and stars revolve. Understanding this, we realize that "the true purpose of all yoga practices is to guide the inner wind out of the side channels and into the central channel." When through the practices of yoga we achieve this, we experience the direct perception of our ultimate reality, and "our body changes from flesh to light."[93]

## Insight about *Chakras* and Points of Stagnation

*Sutra III.29: Nabhi cakre kaya vyuha jnamam.*

> Turn the same effort
> upon the wheel at the navel,
> and you will understand
> the structure of the body.

The relationship and functioning among the two secondary channels and the central channel rely on the abilities of each secondary channel to maintain its respective flow, especially where the intersections of all three meet at specific points known as inner vortexes or wheels (*chakras*). Some authors describe this intersection as a crisscrossing of the secondary channels like twisting vines; when stagnation occurs, it creates choke points on the central channel.[94] Others depict the channels in close proximity without the crossings, implying that

any obstructions are caused by a swelling of the secondary channels when stagnation occurs, reducing the flow of thought energy at
these points.[95] When stagnation or blockages occur at these *chakra*
points, the central channel's ability to maintain its flow and openness
is restricted. This ultimately affects associated physiological centers of
the body (the endocrine glands, nerve plexuses, and organs) in close
proximity to these energetic intersections.

The *chakra* at the navel was the first one to form in the womb, and
it is from there that our entire network of subtle channels and *chakras*
is formed, much as the totality of cells in all the different components
of our physical body formed from the original stem cells of the umbili-
cal cord. Of the seven *chakras*, five are located along the spine (see
figure 4 on page 119). It seems no coincidence that a large percentage
of the physical joint injuries reported in yoga classes, where I suspect
little if any mention is made of the importance of subtle body awareness, are located in proximity to where the subtle body's info-energy
channels and concentrated points of thought-energy meet.

## Insight about the Mind and the Heart

*Sutra III.32–34: Murdha jyotisi siddha darsanam. Pratibhad va sarvam.*
*Hrdaye citta samvit.*

> Turn it upon the radiance
> at the tip of the head,
> and you will see the powers.
> All of them come
> from total understanding.
> Turn it upon the heart,
> and you will know the mind.

For many, the awareness of our *chakra* system begins where subtle
thought-energy stagnates within the subtle channels and produces
sensations of tightness or numbness around them. Working from the
outside in through physical movement and breathing practices and
inside out through meditative practices and intellect requires strong

mental discipline and concerted effort as we progress in discovering the true nature of ourselves and our reality. When we fill our secondary channels with the thoughts of truth and intelligence we have gained through our own life and yogic experience, with genuine empathy for others, we embody what comes naturally as a result: our outer worldly and inner celestial channels (*pingala* and *ida*) are cleared. Then we can open to a fuller experience of divine presence or intelligence in the central channel, which is strongly aligned with the crown *chakra*. With this understanding, we can then turn to the *chakra* of the heart, where "an indestructible drop of consciousness" resides, and where "ultimate love bursts forth with crystal light."[96] It is here that we truly understand the universal nature of our collective minds.

## Insight about Self

*Sutra III.35: Sattva purusayor atyantasamkirnayoh pratyayaviseso bhogh pararthat svartha samyamat purusa jnanam.*

> The causes for reality and the person,
> however very distinct from one another
> these two may be, are no different.
> We experience them not because
> of something outside of ourselves.
> Turn the combined effort upon this,
> and you will understand.

Dealing with the misunderstandings outside of ourselves (reality)—which is the terrain of the sun (masculine) channel—is much simpler than encountering and resolving misunderstandings within ourselves (person)—which inhabits the moon (feminine) channel. Both involve misperception; both situations depend on our mind's interpretation through our five senses to create a label for the "reality" of what we "see" (see figure 3 on page 114). The true reality is only an image (thought-seed) our mind finds, stored among many images programmed into our subconscious.

There is a well-known story in India, retold in the book *How Yoga Works*, in which a teacher of yoga takes a small shoot of bamboo, sharpened at one end, out of a pot of ink on her desk; she holds it up and asks the student what it is.[97] The student automatically replies, "A pen." In a split second, the object seen by the student is determined to be a pen because of its "pen-ness": in other words, the qualities of being a pen that the object possesses are recognized by the student as assumed to be coming from the pen itself. Then the teacher asks the student to follow her outside, where a sacred cow is resting under the shade of a tree. The teacher holds the pen in front of the cow's face and asks the cow what it is. The cow's answer? It starts eating the bamboo. The cow's hunger created a much different answer to what the pen was. How we interpret what we experience depends on our programs, not the object's experience of *itself* by *itself*.

## Insight about Inner and Outer Methods of Yoga

*Sutra I.31: Duhkha daurmanasyangamejayatva svasa prasvasa viksepa sahabhuvah.*

> The mind flies off,
> and with that comes pain in the body;
> unhappy thoughts; shaking in the hands
> and other parts of the body;
> the breath falling out of rhythm
> as it passes in and out.

Coming to understand fully that the complete practice of yoga requires the union of the outer methods (physical postures and breathing practices) with inner methods of meditation and study to illuminate our mental processes, we discover the inseparable interrelationship between our thoughts and our bodies. We become sensitive to the slightest disturbances in the mind that appear in the body (shaking in the hands or other parts; irregular breathing), which in turn cause worry and more disturbance in the mind and more physical symptoms to appear. The beauty of the combination of our outer practices of yoga and the inner work of meditation and study is the wisdom that comes with knowing how the union of those practices can reverse that cycle.

## Insight about Overcoming Obstacles of Incorrect Thinking

*Sutra I.32–33a: Tat pratisedhartham eka tattva abhyasah. Maitri karuna mudita upeksanam sukha duhkha punya apunya vishayanam.*

> And if you wish to stop these obstacles,
> there is one, and only one,
> crucial practice for doing so.
> You must use kindness, compassion, joy, and equanimity.
> Learn to keep your feelings in balance,
> whether something feels good
> or whether it hurts; whether something is enjoyable
> or distasteful.

With consistent practice, we arrive at a place where the slow changes in our personality over years or even decades of practice quicken until we arrive and understand the ultimate importance of thought-energy. Ancient yogis discovered that the three most important psycho-emotional thoughts were kindness, compassion, and joy and that the state of mind those three thoughts naturally produce is equanimity. It is a profound exercise to work toward this and witness the changes slowly taking place within yourself; it is even more powerful to see them manifesting in the lives of people you touch and hold in your thoughts.

## Insight about Correct Thinking and Freedom from Selfishness

*Sutra I.33b–37: Bhavanatas citta prasadanam. Pracchardana vidharanabhyam va pranasya. Visayavati va pravrttirutpanna manasah sthitinibandhani. Visoka va jyotismati. Vitaragavisayam va cittam.*

This practice makes the mind
bright and clear as water.
It gives the same effect as releasing,
then storing, the wind of the breath.
It also helps us control the tendency
that we have, of thoughts constantly arising
about outer objects of experience.
It also makes your heart carefree,
and radiant like starlight.
And it frees your mind from wanting things.

Once we integrate the ultimate importance of thought-energy, there is no turning back. Our mistaken perceptions have been cleansed, and in their place is the direct experience of infinite love. Like the quantum energy of bonding that holds all of creation together, we are beyond human love. The mind is free from needs or wants. All is as it should be, and our purpose is clear: to help and serve others, not in a way that depletes the energy of service and eventually disappears but that inspires and sustains those we help to pursue the same for themselves. This is possible with yoga.

All yoga practitioners should be well-informed
about the functioning of [the subtle body]
because this is the only trustworthy theoretical
foundation for a well-balanced [yoga] practice.

**Shandor Remete**

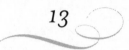

*13*

# *The* Bhutas, Vayus, *and* Marmas

During the first ten years of my yoga practice, the things I learned
about myself were focused primarily on the physical, anatomical
structure of my body. Once I was introduced to the subtler things
that yoga was capable of uncovering, another decade went by, during
which most of what I learned was theoretical. I could see that these
things were possible, but I had a hard time putting them into practice.
When I finally realized that many of the injuries I had accumulated
over years of being a competitive athlete—conditions I felt limited
and, at times, dispirited by—were actually the proving grounds for
these new subtle body concepts, my yoga practice was completely
transformed.

The first step for me was integrating my understanding of *chakras*,
*nadis*, and *koshas* into a framework of movement. From there I looked
to other aspects of the subtle body for guidance. The three components
I discovered to be additionally useful to incorporate while practicing
were *bhutas* (elements), *vayus* (winds), and *marmas* (energy points).
What follows is a simplistic explanation of how to use each of these, as
well as a general framework of where they appear in the body.

# THE *BHUTAS* AND THEIR QUALITIES

In order to achieve perfect physical health, the
ancient sages concluded that you must activate the
body's chakras. Although they possess no physicality,
they govern all the elements of the body.

B. K. S. Iyengar

Each *chakra* is associated with one or more of the specific elements,
also called *bhutas*, that are present in the structure and physical forma-
tion of the human body: earth, water, fire, air, or space/ether. These
elements are manifestations of consciousness that represent different
kinds of energy, and each element is associated with a specific region
of the body. In the practice of physical yoga, what we emphasize mentally through visualization of the subtle qualities of each can create a
stream of psychic-physiological force (*vayus*) that helps energize inner
sensations and keep our presence alive, whether in support of dynamic
movement or static posture.

I have found this extremely helpful, as the mentally imposed muscular effort we rely on for strength, stamina, flexibility, coordination,
control/poise, and balance naturally weakens with age and during
times of limitation due to injury or illness. While practicing, we can
take cues from the properties, qualities, and locations of each element
to intuitively awaken the inner forces they inherently express by feeling
the subtle energetic sensations our elemental thoughts create through
our subtle channels. With practice, we can witness the intuitive muscular or connective tissue response when we surrender ordinary effort.
This provides a sustainable method for maintaining optimal function
and movement at any age.

- **SPACE** (*akasha*): The space that subatomic particles occupy and revolve in; the space found in any hollow area of the body (joints, organs, cavities, pores of the skin). Psychologically, *akasha* can produce feelings of peace, freedom, nonresistance, expansion, and interconnectedness.

- **AIR** (*vayu*): The force that moves electrons around the nucleus; creates flow (of gas, fluid, matter, thought) and vibrations (electrical, psychic) within and beyond the body (such as in the auric perimeter). Psychologically, this can produce feelings of creativity, freshness, vitality, excitation, buoyancy, and clarity.

- **FIRE** (*agni*): The latent or released energy found in atoms; supports metabolic, chemical, and analytical processes in the body (appetite, digestion, body temperature, and assimilation of food, thought, and knowledge). Psychologically, it can produce feelings of determination, stamina, comprehension, absorption, nourishment, transformation, metamorphosis, willpower, appreciation, and warmth.

- **WATER** (*jala*): The bonding energy that keeps protons, neutrons, and electrons attracted to each other; comprises fluids of the body (such as urine, blood, lymph); supports the process of cell hydration. Psychologically, this can produce feelings of softness, empathy, flexibility, love, contentment, cohesion, forgiveness, grace, and coolness.

- **EARTH** (*prithvi*): The dense energy that gives the appearance of matter, substance, stillness, weight, and solidity (for example, protons, neutrons, electrons); comprises the gross matter of the body (bones, teeth, nails, tissues, organs). Psychologically, it can produce feelings of groundedness, support, strength, centeredness, and safety.

| SYMBOL | ELEMENT | LOCATION/REGIONS | TYPES OF ENERGY OR QUALITIES |
|---|---|---|---|
| | Beyond Elements (omnipresent consciousness) | Crown | |
| 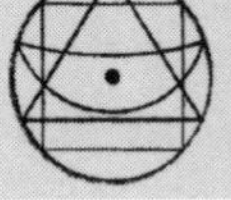 | All Elements (intuition) | Third Eye | |
| • | Space (*Akasha*) | Head/Neck/Throat | subatomic quantum expansive energy |
| 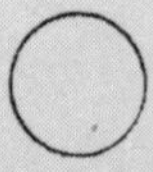 | Air (*Vayu*) | Chest/Thorax | electrical pulsing flow light buoyant energy |
| 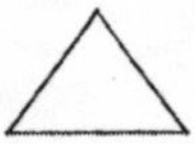 | Fire (*Agni*) | Abdomen/Navel/ Solar Plexus | radiant transforming heating intense energy |
| 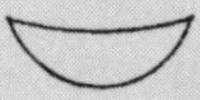 | Water (*Jala*) | Pelvis/Sacrum/Genitals | chemical cleansing cooling soft energy |
| 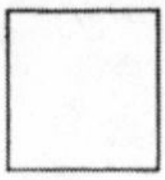 | Earth (*Prithvi*) | Perinreum/Coccyx/Legs/Feet | physical mechanical heavy hard energy |

**FIGURE 6**  The five *bhutas*

# SUBTLE BODY "WINDS"—*VAYUS*

Prana is at work at every instant in every cell of every
living organism, seeking ever to deliver us from
disease and confirm us in health, but only in those
few people who are genetically fated to be healthy does
prana automatically regulate its momentum. The
rest of us must learn how to cultivate our prana.

**Dr. Robert Svoboda**

*Prana*, which means "life force" or "vital energy," can be thought of
as the force that keeps the functions of our bodies animated. It is the
subtle energy that sustains our heart's beating, our lungs' breathing,
and our cells' growth. It is intricately tied to our breathing and is often
misunderstood as air. Although it *is* in the air we breathe, it is more
than air. It is in everything, animate and inanimate; it is a subtle force
operating at submolecular and subatomic levels that forms the basis
of the physical and nonphysical worlds. The early yogis recognized
that *prana* is made up of various components—*vayus* (also known as
"winds")—that are concentrated in different areas of the body and
individually responsible for distinct anatomical and energetic functions. There are ten *vayus* in total, five major (see figure 7 on page 145)
and five minor.

The five major *vayus* (*pranas*) are:

- *Prana vayu*: The outward to inward flow of vital life
  force into the body that enters through the inhale and
  is sent to every cell in our body through the circulatory
  system. *Prana vayu* governs the area below the larynx
  and above the diaphragm and is associated with the
  organs of respiration, sound, and the gullet; it is
  responsible for absorption of atmospheric energy.

- *Samana vayu*: The movement of vital life force from the periphery of the body back to its core, strengthening our body's core vitality, heat-regulating processes, and cell metabolism (e.g., the repair and manufacture of new cells and growth). *Samana vayu* governs the area between the diaphragm and navel and is associated with digestion, assimilation, and the distribution of nutrients.

- *Apana vayu*: The downward and outward flow of vital life force, responsible for the elimination of waste products from the body through the lungs and the moving force behind the exhale. It sustains our excretory systems (genitourinary and gastrointestinal) and is the driving force in the process of reproduction (i.e., moving new life out into the world). *Apana vayu* governs the area below the navel into the pelvic floor and is associated with the organs of elimination, ejaculation, and childbirth.

- *Udana vayu*: The upward and outward movement of vital life force responsible for speech and expelling air with exhalation in a way that is particularly concerned with sound production through the vocal apparatus (i.e., speaking, singing, laughing, and crying). It also governs vomiting, nausea, and coughing. *Udana vayu* governs the area above the base of the throat and activates all of the sensory receptors of the nose, mouth, eyes, and ears. It also assists with balance and movement of the limbs.

- *Vyana vayu*: The movement of *prana* from the chest center out to the periphery; it is associated with the cardiovascular system. *Vyana vayu* pervades the whole body and is a connecting force responsible for subtle movement and coordination throughout the whole organism. It also acts as a reserve force for all the other *vayus*.

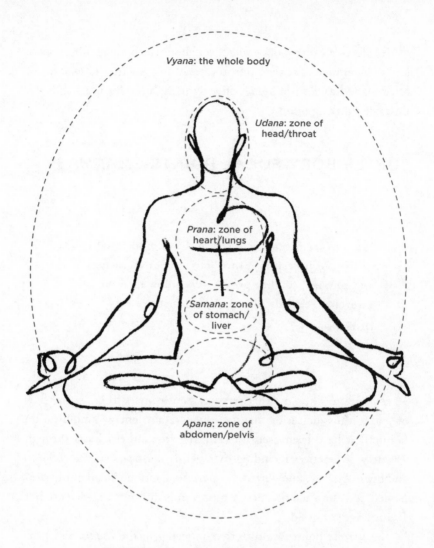

Vyana: the whole body

Udana: zone of
head/throat

Prana: zone of
heart/lungs

Samana: zone
of stomach/
liver

Apana: zone of
abdomen/pelvis

**FIGURE 7** The subtle body *vayus* (*pranas*)

The five minor *vayus* (*upapranas*) are *naga* (responsible for belching and hiccups), *kurma* (controls blinking and the iris, which regulates the intensity of light for sight), *krikara* (generates thirst, hunger, sneezing, and coughing), *devadatta* (induces sleep and yawning), and *dhananjaya* (produces phlegm and lingers immediately after death to decompose the body).

To effectively distribute *prana* throughout the body requires a calm and stable mind. To achieve this, the breathing practices of *pranayama* are designed to control *prana*, offering us stability for our habitually unstable thinking mind.

## SUBTLE BODY FOCAL POINTS—*MARMAS*

Marmas are portals into the multi-dimensionality of life. As junction points between consciousness and physiology, they provide a window into the interchangeability of energy and matter.

**David Simon**

*Marmas* are focal points that serve as transformers to boost the flow of *prana*, thus increasing vitality. They are also energy-amplification points that have been used for centuries in southern India through a variety of practices including therapeutic massage (*marma chikitsa*) and the martial art known as *kalaripayattu*, a unique blend of physical, mental, and spiritual practices whose aim is not only self-defense but also strength of mind.

The *marma* points are directly connected to the *chakra* and *nadi* systems and facilitate the circulation of vital life-force energy all over the body. Manipulating them can balance energy within *chakras* and increase flow through the *nadis*. *Marma* points produce local effects in the regions where they are and "stimulate, pacify, or balance aspects of the mind and body near and far away."[98]

## Marmas, Bhutas, and Regions of the Body

The body can be divided into five regions, each relating to one of the five *bhutas*. We can balance the properties of our body's elements by working with the *marmas* in the region that relates to them.

- *Marmas* in the region of the feet belong to
  the earth element. This region's key *marma* is
  *talhridaya*, located in the soles of the feet.

- *Marmas* in the region from the knees to the anus
  belong to the water element. This region's key *marma*
  is *urvi*, located in the middles of the thighs.

- *Marmas* in the region from the anus to the
  heart belong to the fire element. This area's
  key *marma* is *nabhi*, located in the navel.

- *Marmas* in the region from the heart to the middle
  of the eyebrows belong to the air element. The
  key *marma* here is *phana*, found in the nostrils.

- *Marmas* in the region from the middle of the eyebrows to the
  top of the head belong to the ether element. The key *marma*
  in this area is *adhipati*, located on the apex of the head.

In *hatha* yoga practice, we can make use of *marma* points as gateways into the *nadis* and *chakras* of the subtle body, as well as links into the systems of the gross physical body, such as the cardiovascular, neuromuscular, endocrinological, and immunological systems. We can also activate the *marmas* through an ancient form of *pratyahara* (often translated as "control" or "withdrawal" of the senses) and *dharana* (a type of meditation with single-pointed focus). The classical yoga text *Vasistha Samhita* states, "A meditator should practice meditation [*dharana*] only after being distinctly cognizant [by drawing one's *prana* by the power of attention] of the vital spots in the body [*marma* points], the system of *nadis* [channels], places and functions of the *vayus* [*pranas*]."[99]

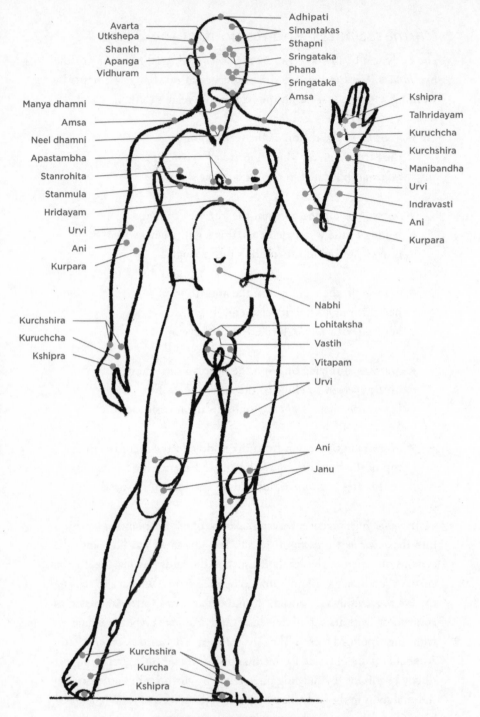

**FIGURE 8A** Subtle body *marmas*

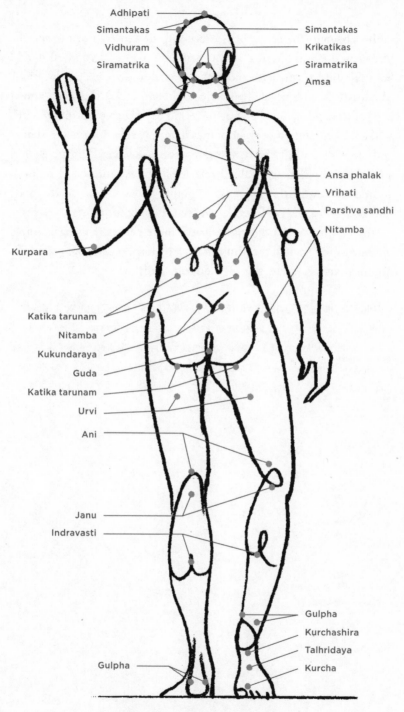

**FIGURE 8B** Subtle body *marmas*

Labels, top left: Adhipati, Simantakas, Vidhuram, Siramatrika

Labels, top right: Simantakas, Krikatikas, Siramatrika, Amsa

Labels, right: Ansa phalak, Vrihati, Parshva sandhi, Nitamba

Labels, left: Kurpara

Labels, lower left: Katika tarunam, Nitamba, Kukundaraya, Guda, Katika tarunam, Urvi, Ani, Janu, Indravasti, Gulpha

Labels, lower right: Gulpha, Kurchashira, Talhridaya, Kurcha

It is beyond the scope of this book to describe all of the specific *marma* points and the areas they control, but figures 8A and 8B should help familiarize you with most of the well-known *marma* locations. Much as I do with my daily practice of *asana*, I use the general knowledge of how subtle body energy moves in each yoga pose and gravity's influence on familiar *marma* points to intuitively inform the shapes and movement of my body. On rare occasions when I intuitively feel something is off energetically, I refer to the illustrations and seek out additional information on specific points and the areas of the body they control (see LEVITYoGA.com/subtle-body for more resources).

You can start working with *marmas* more generally using a simple method of intentional breathing at each region's key *marma* points. To do this practice, follow this method mindfully:

SITTING STILL IN A COMFORTABLE POSITION AND BREATHING THROUGH THE NOSE, slowly inhale, with your full attention and sense of presence, into the key point in each region, one at a time, psychically "touching" it with the fullness of your breath. With each exhale, soften and surrender completely into the sensations around the key point as you feel the inner void that your departing breath creates. Visualize your fullest healing potential taking its place.

# PART 5

## Practice Essentials

I have things in my head that are not like what anyone
has taught me—shapes and ideas so near to me—so
natural to my way of being and thinking . . . I decided
to start anew, to strip away what I had been taught.

**Georgia O'Keeffe**

In the February 1999 issue of *Yoga Journal*, six well-known Western
yoga teachers from six different styles of yoga were asked to provide
written tutorials for six common yoga poses, describing the "correct"
techniques necessary to perform each pose.[100] The editors arranged
the teachers' descriptions side by side, accompanied with photos of
each pose modeled by each teacher's top student. The pictures were
identically formatted—using the same camera angle, backdrop, and
lighting—giving readers a comprehensive overview of each style's take
on a pose.

At first glance, you could see that all the photos for a particular pose
were similar, though some physical differences stood out. Reading each
teacher's narrative about how to "do" and "be" in a pose highlighted
the contrasts in technique even more.

Not obvious or explicitly revealed in the article was the fact that all but two of the teachers and styles selected had descended from the same lineage of a legendary sage and yoga master from Chennai, India, named Tirumalai Krishnamacharya. Until his death in 1989 at the age of 100, Krishnamacharya had concentrated his efforts on adapting, and in many ways revolutionizing, yogic practice for the modern world. He was known as a generous, though often intense, teacher who was dedicated to teaching to the individual, always adapting to the unique set of circumstances of each student. His top pupils were many of the greatest exponents of yoga to the West and produced a generation of Indian and Western teachers, including his son, T. K. V. Desikachar, as well as B. K. S. Iyengar, Indra Devi, and K. Pattabhi Jois. These four teachers went on to create their own styles of yoga, with distinctly different approaches to its practice, and were mostly responsible for the modern popularization of yoga outside of India.[101]

In particular, Iyengar and Jois established stylized systems of yoga (Iyengar and Ashtanga, respectively) that became extremely popular in the United States and Europe, producing thousands of teachers to carry the torch of Krishnamacharya's lineage to a growing population of global yoga enthusiasts. These two men played a huge role in transforming the physical practices of *hatha* yoga, seen traditionally as a preliminary part of yoga's eight-limb process of self-discovery, into a more primary role for initiating a Western mind-set and lifestyle into yoga.

When the article was published, Iyengar yoga was all I knew yoga to be. As a student and teacher, I was continually reminded how "dangerous" it would be to wander from Iyengar's teachings: that it would create confusion if students borrowed ideas from other styles of yoga. Nevertheless, those *Yoga Journal* photographs challenged me intellectually. It was probably the first time I seriously questioned what I had been taught; I found myself asking whether other possibilities existed on my yogic path. If nothing else, the article aroused my curiosity.

As it happened, a yoga teacher new to town showed up early one morning for class and, afterward, asked if she could teach Ashtanga yoga at our studio. I had heard about this style while in India but knew practically nothing of it. With the article fresh in my mind and without much thought, I said yes, though with one condition: that she would teach me.

Although I continued to teach Iyengar yoga, my practice for the next two years was the flowing, ever-moving elegance of Ashtanga. I was fascinated with the differences between these two styles and the dissimilar physical and psychological effects they produced in me. But, as Iyengar had warned, this period also brought confusion. How could two accomplished teachers of the same master in India produce such uniquely different forms of yoga? What was it about the way Krishnamacharya taught that allowed his top disciples to move beyond what they had learned with him to create and teach dramatically different personal styles of yoga? Answering those questions became a greater passion for me than just learning another style.

## LEGACY AND LINEAGE

In his book *Health, Healing, and Beyond*, Desikachar describes his father's most enduring contribution as:

> [The] ability to express the theory and practice of yoga
> in concrete, practical terms . . . discarding even the most
> sanctified past teaching if he felt that it was unclear or
> unhelpful. He chose aspects of yoga that he found through
> trial and error to be the most suitable in the modern world.
> Krishnamacharya's task was to bring all that he knew into a
> coherent system.[102]

According to an article on Krishnamacharya's legacy, "While he had enormous respect for the past, he also didn't hesitate to experiment and innovate. By developing and refining different approaches, he made yoga accessible to millions."[103]

As diverse as the methods and knowledge of Krishnamacharya's lineage have become, passion and faith in yoga remain their common heritage, along with creativity and innovation. The tacit message found in its history over generations is that "yoga is not a static tradition—it's a living, breathing art that grows constantly through each practitioner's experiments and deepening experience."[104] I was beginning to see what lay ahead and that the teachers who had come before me—Krishnamacharya,

Iyengar, and Shandor—possessed all four of these traits. I felt fortunate to share them as well. If I were able to apply what I had learned so far through the practice and teaching of yoga into a form that was approachable for anyone interested in yoga, what would be the most effective way to offer it? How could I meet students where they were in life and provide guidance toward authenticity without undue influence—without robbing them of their own experience by handing them a list of poses and the "expected" results from practice?

It became clear I was not to create just another style of yoga with "newer" techniques and join a "yoga-fitness" industry oversaturated with styles and brands. Instead, I saw a need for a simpler approach to yogic principles that could prepare students for the ultimate solo journey—toward the inner teacher we all embody.

My role in the process was to record the insights that were revealed to me in clear, straightforward language. Then, as a teacher, I could step back and look for ways to reduce what I had to its bare essence and see whether what was left fit together. My goal was to create a guide that students could use to go beyond what they had learned so far and arrive at their own understanding of yoga, supported by a lineage whose traditions encouraged them to do so.

This process took time—decades, really—testing the language I used to convey what had become the essential elements of my practice to create a vocabulary that could "cross borders" and be received by yoga students from any style. I consolidated and arranged the elements into three principles of practice, which you can apply at any level of ability to any style of yoga to create *conscious movement*, especially when experiencing limitations in mobility due to injury or preexisting conditions.

## PRACTICE PRINCIPLES

I conceived the following Practice Principles to guide you creatively in establishing a personal practice by meeting yourself where you find yourself on a daily basis, physically and psychologically. They rely only on your ability to be present with whatever shows up when practicing and to engage—to be in relationship with the now of your experience and work with what you have in that moment.

Together, the three Practice Principles help you:

- Recognize and eliminate unnecessary effort in your practice

- Reduce external distractions

- Discover facile, less-obvious catalysts for movement

The principles are intentionally vague in terms of musculoskeletal technique. Instead, applying these basic principles helps you direct attention toward points or areas of your body where resistance is present and movement is limited. These places offer the clearest guidance for what is necessary to create or restore balance; when approached with renewed awareness, they allow you to feel the influence that focused attention and proper breathing have to effect change and healing.

Embracing all three principles during practice helps you minimize physically overworking the poses and allows any pose to naturally activate the body-mind response that the inherent shape of the pose offers. This approach prepares you to experience new or unfamiliar physical sensations in your body without psychological distress. It strengthens your intuitive ability to adjust in the present to any pose and prepares you to develop more intimacy with the experiences on your mat—to interpret messages and language the body uses to communicate what's needed in any situation.

As you understand and master the Practice Principles, you develop new ways for working safely and efficiently, guiding you toward a truly personal practice with the authority of your inner teacher. The three principles are:

- Back-Body Breathing

- Spine Mechanics

- Fundamentals of Flow

In the remaining three chapters, we will explore these in order.

Feelings come and go like clouds in a windy sky. Conscious breathing is my anchor.

**Thich Nhat Hanh**

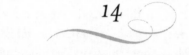

# Back-Body Breathing

Generally, we learn how to breathe without any training, and by the time we're adults, limited patterns of breathing that unconsciously reduce our lungs' natural capacity are firmly established neurologically. We are told "good" breathing means filling our belly with breath so the abdominal wall distends and the full lung is accessed. This is often referred to as yogic or belly breathing. Typically, the primary orientation where we experience our breath is forward, into the frontal domain of the lungs. When employing the principle of Back-Body Breathing, however, the orientation of the breath shifts, redirecting the physical breath to more fully access the back and sides of the lungs.

## ORIENTATION OF BREATH

When we consciously inhale, we experience the physical sensation of our lungs expanding. As the lungs expand, other musculoskeletal processes occur. Most of us can simultaneously feel the frontal rib cage expanding ever so slightly. Less obvious is feeling the expansion of the skin and muscle tissue covering our ribs. What's even less obvious—until we place attention into our backs—is feeling the three-dimensional expansion of ribs, skin, and muscle tissue: front, side, and back. As we breathe with attention placed into our backs, we can feel the influence the expanding back-body has on the spine. Initially, the movement of the spine with breath is so remote that you may not perceive the spine moving at all.

But like much of the work we employ to connect with the subtle body, we can use the mind to visualize movement in the spine based on what we *expect* to find until the neural pathways are established to the point where physical sensation is created and feels "real." Visualization can trick parts of the brain that directly affect the response in our nervous system into neurologically experiencing what we imagine.[105] There are many examples of how this works in modern life (reacting to a dramatic movie and the placebo effect both come to mind).

Back-Body Breathing is the first principle to learn as a beginner; it starts with one of the simplest and oldest poses our bodies know, Child's Pose (*Balasana*), shown in figure 9.

This pose is taught in a variety of ways, but for the purpose of reorienting your breath, knees touching each other is best, with your arms back alongside the legs. In this variation, your thighs compress the belly and frontal ribs, provoking a confrontation with typical front-body breathing; realignment of the breath is a natural outcome of the shape of the pose. By inhibiting the habit of front-body breathing, you create a more even distribution of breath to access underutilized terrain in the back and side lobes of the lung; this has beneficial effects on both your physiology and psychology.

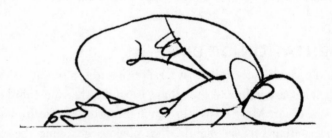

**FIGURE 9** Child's Pose (*Balasana*)

It is a misconception that typical "belly breathing," where the abdominal wall bloats outward, is best for the abdominal organs. With practice in Child's Pose, you can see how learning to restrain the navel slightly as you inhale gently compresses your internal organs, which increases the peristaltic pressure that occurs naturally when the diaphragm is pressed down. Think of it as self-massage for your internal organs, gently squeezing them against a stationary abdominal wall by the flattening of the diaphragm as you inhale and liberating them fully when the diaphragm releases and retreats as you exhale.

**TO EXPERIENCE BACK-BODY BREATHING IN CHILD'S POSE,** kneel down and fold forward into Child's Pose, with your feet and knees together, touching. Initially, you may feel shortness of breath, so be creative with modifications. (If needed, bring your arms forward, partially supporting the weight of your torso with your forearms and resting your head on a foam block or folded blanket.) Consciously slow your breath: a three- to four-second inhale and a three- to four-second exhale. With each inhale, move your attention with the sensation of your breath: from your nostrils into the nasal passages down into the back of the throat, back of the heart, back of the belly, back of the pelvis, and into the pelvic floor. With each exhale, soften where the belly and ribs meet your thighs and feel the weight of your internal organs falling. Soften the collarbones and feel the weight of your shoulders falling. Soften deep into your hip creases (where the tops of your legs meet your pelvis) and feel your torso heavy on your thighs.

At each cycle of breath, feel the subtle expansion of the lungs as you inhale, spreading the skin across your back for the full length of your torso; on the exhale, soften where the belly and ribs meet your thighs, and feel gravity pressing you flatter onto the legs, occasionally sliding your head forward on the floor as your spine naturally lengthens. After five cycles of breath, come out of the pose with an inhale.

Anatomically, as you learn to fully release the connective tissue around the abdominal and thoracic organs and intercostal spaces of your rib cage, a subtle internal sensation of "space" is created as you feel the weight of your organs sinking. This awareness helps develop more capacity for breathing. With consistent practice, releasing subconscious contraction in the diaphragm, intercostal muscle, and connective tissue, the paraspinal muscles of the back are simultaneously released and your spine naturally lengthens, providing even more free-dom for breathing.

Emphasizing Back-Body Breathing helps you cultivate deeper sen-sitivity to subtle sensations and is one of the gateways to the energetic systems of the subtle body. By keeping your awareness with the sensa-tion of your breath into the back-body, you experience the breath's subtle influence on spinal movement, which subsequently stimulates movement of sensation into the energy points and channels of the subtle body.

To see a more detailed explanation and graphical representation of the subtle body components found in this pose, refer to "Subtle Body Guidesheet 1" in the appendix.

## PHYSICAL BREATH VS. SUBTLE BREATH

Our physical breath supports the physiological processes we depend on for all our biological functioning. The action of breathing delivers oxygen into our lungs, which transfers to the blood, is transported to our cells, and provides what is needed to oxidize food. We learn very early in life that exercise is healthy because it produces a very efficient cardiovascular transfer to keep our physical bodies nourished and in optimum balance.

Our yogic ancestors discovered that when they controlled the physical breath, it provided more than just physical nourishment and health. Their practices also allowed access to new states of being and awareness, as well as the realization that we are more than just physi-cal bodies and that breath provides more than just physical breath. They referred to these more refined and subtle aspects of breathing as *prana* ("subtle breath").

Particularly relevant to the practice of yoga is how the subtle breath and physical breath work together. A beautiful analogy is that of a boat moving swiftly across a calm lake, producing a wake in its path. The physical breath, like the boat, is propelled by a physical force as the diaphragm and intercostal muscles of the ribs engage and release. Subtle breath, like the wake, is dependent on the physi-cal breath but sustains its own independent momentum and gentle movement and can be modified wherever we place our attention, much as the wake of the boat is influenced by the wind or tides.

This principle is also found in the martial art practice of qigong, where *qi* ("life force," "vital breath") follows *yi* ("mind's attention," "consciousness"). In yoga, *prana Shakti* ("life force," "subtle breath") follows *chitta Shakti* ("mind's attention or consciousness"). This gives us the ability to use the physical breath and our minds together to direct the subtle breath where we place our attention and to invigorate places in our bodies and minds where we feel stuck or congested.

## QUALITIES OF BREATH

Pranayama is mostly a practice for the ears, and of listening.
B. K. S. Iyengar

Breathing practices (*pranayama*) that the ancient yogis discovered were known to establish an optimum natural, physical breath for a healthy body and produce psychological states to reduce stress and improve mental clarity. More advanced techniques were found to increase levels of perception beyond the physical and psychological sense of self and were capable of creating heightened states of awareness superior to the individual body-mind, into deep meditation and further, into a realm described as "divine bliss" (*samadhi*).

Many schools of yoga suggest that *pranayama* should only be undertaken with the guidance of an experienced teacher, to avoid unexpected and potentially harmful reactions to its powerful influence on the subtle aspects of mind and body. To ensure a safe practice of *pranayama*, recommendations are given for observing various ethical lifestyle choices (*yamas*); maintaining a healthy diet, regular hygiene, sufficient rest, and study (*niyamas*); and doing a consistent practice of physical postures (*asana*). Numerous old yoga texts warn that unless body afflictions and disease are eliminated prior to practicing *pranayama*, more serious conditions could arise. Here another paradox presents itself: Which comes first—practices to create an open body, physically and psychologically, that allow the safe practice of refined states of conscious breathing, or practices of conscious breathing that assist the safe opening of the body through the practice of *asana*? As with most paradoxes, it's a little of both.

I recommend students begin conscious breathing in their very first practice using a rudimentary technique of noticing three simple qualities of breath—*sound, rhythm,* and *texture*. There are important reasons for this. At the most basic level, conscious breathing requires present-moment awareness, where the mind is trained to stay fully in the present. Breath is one of the most useful tools for achieving this. Also, our breath is a window into the subconscious, where disturbances in the mind can show up initially as disturbances in the breath. With proficiency in controlling these three qualities of breath, a natural balance arises in the mind, which improves our ability to remain calm under any circumstance. With the wisdom and stillness calm brings, you can incorporate other practices with the subtle breath.

## Sound

Breath has a dualistic relationship with many parts of our central nervous system. The sympathetic branch of our autonomic nervous system has the ability to subconsciously change our breathing as needed to prepare for stressful situations (think scary movies or, if you're a parent, driving for the first time with your teenager). In the opposite way, the breath has the ability to change our parasympathetic nerve response to naturally defuse stress (think of sighing or when your nine-year-old daughter says, "Take a breath, Dad"). Sound is a simple way to monitor and control the rhythm of your breath.

So, begin your breathing practice with the sound of the breath. Naturally, when breathing through the nose we typically hear the sound of air moving through the nostrils, especially when we're breathing heavily or our nasal passages are congested. The first practice is to *take control of this sound* and shift it into the throat. Imagine the sound you make when forcefully exhaling through the mouth. Try it: it creates a subtle contraction of muscles at the back of the throat (glottis vocalis), and the air that passes through this slightly restricted area produces a raspy sound and subtle vibration in the tissues of the oral cavity. With practice, you can create this contraction with your mouth closed and make the same sound while both inhaling and exhaling through the nose (known as *ujjayi* breath).

Once you produce the proper sound, you can learn to control its pitch. The optimum pitch for the parasympathetic nerves is a sound that is soft and low, like a whisper audible only to yourself. If the pitch increases and becomes hard and high, it produces an aggressive sound, commonly referred to in the average yoga class as "Darth Vader breath," which often triggers a sympathetic nerve response, causing an aggressive response in the body.

## Rhythm

The next step to conscious breathing is to control the rhythm of the breath and return its tempo to a more natural pace, the one we entered life with. It is a common misconception that deep breathing is the most beneficial breath, especially if it is forced with imposed muscular effort. But merely slowing the breath has been shown to be the most effective way to stimulate the vagus nerve, which is a primary activator of the parasympathetic response for calming and relaxation. It also trains the nervous system to prepare for the more advanced practices of subtle body contractions (*bandhas*) at the root, belly, and throat subtle body energy centers (*chakras*).

After the age of four, our unconscious breath as we go about our day averages a one- to two-second inhale and an even shorter exhale. To begin creating a slower rhythm, start with a three- to four-second inhale followed by a three- to four-second exhale. For the first few rounds, internally count to yourself, until you familiarize yourself, through sound, with the tempo of your breath. This practice seems simple, and when you're practicing slow moving or still poses, it is. Challenge yourself by practicing slow breathing when moving dynamically during a vigorous practice. Before you realize it, you will be able to control the rhythm of your breath with any pace of activity. This becomes a valuable skill for the more advanced *pranayama* practices of breath retention and alternate nostril breathing, which require an ability to separate the physical and psychological parts of breathing and literally control the need to breathe.

## Texture

When you consistently control the breath, it is easier to create a smooth, even rhythm for the amounts of time spent inhaling and exhaling. Simultaneously, if you maintain a soft sound with the breath, you begin to notice a recognizable breath texture. Look particularly at the transitions that cycle between inhalation and exhalation, and exhalation and inhalation. Texture defines the consistency, or lack thereof, in the sound of the breath. Ideally the sound should be free of fluctuation and smooth as silk. If too much effort is employed to control either sound or rhythm, the texture of the breath suffers. Go with the flow and don't overextend your capacities when controlling the breath; rest when you need to and try again later. Notice whether one phase of the breath is easier than the other. If inhalations are easier to slow down and extend (exhalations being more challenging), consciously extend your inhalations even longer. If exhalations are easier to slow down and extend (inhalations being more challenging), consciously extend your exhalations even longer. These impositions on the stronger cycle of breath will assist the weaker cycles in lengthening and strengthening.

With this simple foundation of breathing exercises using the three qualities of sound, rhythm, and texture, your practice of *asana* will achieve a higher level of presence for safer movement.

## PHASES OF BREATHING

Another practice for refining the breath is recognizing that each phase of breathing has different properties that contribute unique opportunities to experience poses more intimately and effortlessly. The phases of the breath are *inhalation, exhalation,* and *retention.* By working with the unique aspects of each phase, an intimate relationship with discomfort arises that helps transform uncomfortable encounters with physical and psychological imbalance in the muscles, joints, and connective tissues of the body. This, in turn, increases the effectiveness of the subtle breath for rewiring the neurological response when moving into poses that produce unpleasant sensations (resistance).

### Inhalation (*Puraka*)

As I mentioned before, when we inhale, the physical breath fills the lungs, and we can feel the sensation of the expanding lung. To feel the subtle breath while inhaling, start by visualizing the inflating lung gently expanding into the ribs (front, side, and back), then into the skin covering the ribs, and ultimately moving into and along the spine. When this practice produces a true experience of subtle sensation moving within, you can use this technique throughout the body anywhere you place your attention.

Now try a simple experiment:

SIT COMFORTABLY ON THE FLOOR WITH YOUR LEGS CROSSED. Close your eyes. Place your attention with your physical breath. As you slowly inhale, notice the skin at the tip of your nostrils cooling as the incoming air moves past. Follow the cool sensation from the nostrils up into the nasal passages of the head, feeling the cool and subtle expansion against the nasal linings, then down into the back of your throat, the back of your heart, the back of your kidneys, the back of your rectum, and into the pelvic floor. As your breath reaches the pelvic floor, feel the skin across your buttocks, hips, and perineum expand slightly. If you don't immediately feel movement, visualize the skin in each location spreading with your breath until you do. Be patient. This process takes time and consistent practice.

Cooling and expansion are the two primary subtle energies of inhalation. The energy of cooling reduces heat and is useful for areas of the body and mind that have been overworked through repetitive strain (think how effective ice packs are for inflammation or headache symptoms). The energy of expansion helps create awareness in the fullness of our being: physical, mental, and emotional. It is the ebb cycle of breathing and movement, like a retreating wave that is drawn back into the fullness of the ocean. Physically, we use this phase to exit poses gracefully. Psychologically, we use this phase to mitigate anxiety when approaching our edge, letting the subtle expansion of the breath slightly lift us out of a pose, giving our physical body a pause and our mind a calming experience, as though we were finished with the pose and coming out of it. This produces a reboot for our nervous system to reacquaint itself with the situation and adjust, knowing that we have the ability to determine our tolerance for meeting resistance with each cycle of breath.

With each inhale, using your attention and breath at will to create subtle sensation throughout the body gives you a powerful tool for meeting both physical and psychological tenderness or grip, as well as any neurological sensitivity stored in various locations of the body.

## Exhalation (*Rechaka*)

When we exhale, the physical breath empties the lungs, and we can feel the sensation of the deflating lung. To feel the subtle breath exhaling, start by visualizing the energy of the breath as a warm softness from the pelvis, exiting into the organs of the abdomen, the diaphragm, the lungs, and the throat. This sensation produces an internal experience of space and profound relaxation, even where chronic tension exists. When this practice produces a true experience of warm softness and the freedom it creates, you can use it throughout the body, anywhere you place your attention.

**TO HAVE A LITTLE EXPERIENCE OF THIS,** lie down with your back flat on the floor, as comfortably as you can (use a bolster or other support under your thighs or head as needed). Close your eyes. Place your attention with your physical breath. With each slow inhale, follow the sensation of your breath from the nostrils through the back-body and the full length of your torso, as if the floor were part of your lungs. As you slowly exhale, notice the skin warming at your nostrils' aperture as the outgoing air moves past.

Consciously soften the top of your lungs and feel the weight of your heart dropping. Soften the diaphragm, feel the weight of your abdominal organs dropping; soften the sphincter muscles, feel the weight of your genitals dropping; soften the front of your throat, feel the weight of the thyroid gland dropping. With each exhale, as you feel the front-body softening and the weight of your internal organs dropping, simultaneously feel gravity pressing you flatter into the floor and the spine passively lengthening. Extend your head slightly as you feel your neck naturally lengthening.

Warming and softness are the two primary subtle energies of exhalation. The energy of warming assists with relaxation, stimulates circulation, and is useful for areas of the body and mind that are chronically tight (think how effective hot water bottles are for chronic tension in the body or for reducing coldness due to lack of circulation). The energy of softness helps create a feeling of more internal space in our being—physically, mentally, and emotionally. It is the flow cycle of breathing, like an advancing ocean wave that washes onto the beach. Physically, we use this phase to enter poses effortlessly, employing gravity and its effects as a catalyst for movement into the spaces we create with softness. Psychologically, we use this phase to build intuition and the ability to respond to an invitation to move created in the moment of surrender. This is a safer way to move into poses, released from the greed of mentally imposed, muscular effort to "achieve" a final shape of the pose. With each cycle of breath, we always have the ability to surrender a little more to things as they are and move into the space we create.

With each exhale, using your attention and breath at will to create subtle softness throughout the body gives you a powerful tool for meeting both physical and psychological hardness or anxiety, as well as any neurological stagnation stuck in various locations of the body.

## Retention (*Kumbhaka*)

In yoga, breath retention practices are powerful ways to build mental energy and create deep inner tranquility and poise. Mastering breath retentions involves a series of slow and patient practices that take years to develop, involving preliminary periods of deep relaxation and stillness, in comfortable seated or supine (flat on your back) poses. Retention practices can be a form of meditation by themselves, or they can be integrated into the practice of individual yoga poses or dynamic sequences.

**AS A MEDITATION,** start with a comfortable position and consciously slow your breath until you have established an effortless three- to four-second inhale and three- to four-second exhale. Doing nasal breathing for each phase, keep the sound of your breath (*ujjayi*) soft and the texture of your breath smooth. After an initial four to five rounds of breathing, change to a rhythm of six- to eight-second inhales and six- to eight-second exhales.

After four to five rounds, when you have settled into an effortless rhythm, again change the rhythm, aiming for ten- to twelve-second inhales and ten- to twelve-second exhales. At whatever level your breath reaches for your longest duration with effortless rhythm, stay there for another four to five cycles of breath.

When you reach the last exhalation on the last cycle, slowly initiate the next inhale until you're comfortably full (don't overinflate) and hold your breath (inhalation retention). As you hold the breath, consciously soften your diaphragm and feel your abdominal organs sink a little. Gently swallow once. Re-release your diaphragm if it contracted during the swallow. Hold your breath as long as you can without anxiety. If you feel any anxiety rising, try swallowing and re-releasing the diaphragm again to retain the breath a little longer.

When you need to, slowly exhale and resume breathing with whatever rhythm the breath naturally finds, without effort. Breathe like this for four to five rounds.

You can repeat this same practice for exhalation retentions.

Breath retention helps concentrate mental energy while simultaneously withdrawing energy from the sense organs and turning your attention inward. It creates a state of being where time and outside concerns dissolve. It changes brain activity, slowing the frequency of neurological impulses and producing deep calm and contentment. It also provides a glimpse of the frontier that separates life and death and builds an appreciation of living in the moment and gratitude for the life you have.

## MASTERY OF SUBTLE BODY BREATHING

Each cycle of the breath has unique properties that can aid in experiencing unfamiliar physical sensations and psychological states of being in your poses. This occurs as you understand that all movement is preceded by consciousness, and all sensation and thought you experience result in both conscious and subconscious neuromuscular response.

With mastery of subtle body breathing, you can use your movement, your mind, and your breath as effective pain management tools, empowering yourself and reclaiming the inner authority for your life. Subtle body breathing is also extremely useful as your physical practice of poses deepens, giving you a safe way to overcome or integrate resistance to movement. There is nothing magical to be found in our poses if conscious breathing is absent. With consistent practice of Back-Body Breathing, we slowly develop an intimate relationship with the qualities of the breath and our ability to apply them to create physical and psychological balance in our lives.

The body is designed to distribute
strain globally, not to focus it locally.

**Thomas Myers and James Earls**

## 15

# Spine Mechanics

In one way or another, the spine is intricately involved in all yoga poses.
The reasons for this are many. The first masters of yoga understood the
critical role the spine plays in supporting the body's vital processes,
and movement of the spine through *asana* promotes its healthy function and the physical body's overall health. They also discovered latent
forces in the spine that awaken capacities of the body beyond the physical and came to recognize the physical body as just the outer layer of
numerous bodies within. (See "The *Koshas*" in chapter 9.)

Among the almost infinite number of yoga poses, each shape has
distinct influences to support the spine's ability to function in eight
unique directions: forward and back bending; left and right side
bending; left and right spinal rotation (twisting); extension and compression. Of the eight, only compression is actively discouraged in
*hatha* yoga, although anatomically this common, functional restric-
tion of the spine is another one of the mysterious paradoxes found in
the practice; a little bit of compression is not only good but also necessary for circulation and bone density in a healthy spine. The range
of movement these eight directions provide stimulates, supplies, and

circulates blood to the brain and spinal cord and promotes the health of the tissues rooted there.

Many teachers of yoga and structural anatomy focus on the unique properties and function of the spine in its parts (cervical, thoracic, lumbar, sacral, and coccyx) without a holistic understanding of the spine's design and its full, nearly boundless potential in creating movement in three-dimensional space to accommodate the wide variety of yoga poses that are available. Numerous medical doctors, orthopedic surgeons, and chiropractors I have spoken with believe many yoga poses—especially those where the body simultaneously engages multiple directions of movement—are anatomically unsafe for the spine, such as twisting while simultaneously back bending. To support their claims, they often cite the number of yoga-related back and neck injuries they treat in their offices.

For many students of yoga (and not just beginners), dealing with acute or chronic pain from minor back injury is inevitably a part of life—and is lately becoming more a part of yoga classes, where the reported number of class-related injuries is on the rise. In 2009, the *International Journal of Yoga Therapy* published a report that investigated yoga class injury types, severity, frequency, associated poses, and other factors. Injuries of the neck and lower back were consistently near the top in type, severity, and frequency. The study cited "poor technique or alignment, previous injury, excess effort, and improper or inadequate instruction" as the most common causes of yoga-related injuries, and it left little doubt that injuries are increasingly common. According to the authors, "injuries that occur from participating in classes at the very least, impair the true experience of Yoga"; but more than that, "such instances can lead to serious injury, permanent disability, and even death."[106]

Of the top factors that are likely to cause injury, the students' and teachers' lack of yoga experience or knowledge plays a major role. Many of the reasons students are getting hurt point to the responsibility of the teacher: improper instruction or sequencing; lack of instruction or warm-up; peer pressure (from fellow students or a teacher); class size (meaning lack of teacher attention toward students or lack of student connection/trust with teacher); and undisclosed (intentionally or unintentionally) preexisting conditions. What wasn't mentioned in the study was the style of yoga being practiced when an injury occurred; it simply implied that all styles of yoga are created equal. They are not, especially when it comes to injuries. A student's decision to attend a yoga class, injured or not, is rarely informed by the therapeutic effects of various styles of yoga or the depth of a teacher's experience; it often has more to do with teacher or class popularity and/or the convenience of a studio's location or schedule.

If you are injured or have limited mobility and are new to practicing yoga, appropriate movement depends on an experienced teacher, preferably one with firsthand experience of physical limitations and the challenges that come with each phase of healing: sometimes requiring rest; at other times, mindful and effortful movement. For back injuries especially, a thorough understanding of what supports healthy movement in the spine—anatomically and energetically—is necessary at different stages of healing. The fundamentals of Spine Mechanics will give you a basic understanding of your spine's potential in its current state of health and provide the tools for achieving your optimum movement. With consistent practice, this approach has the power to safely create a greater range of motion, flexibility, strength, and overall health for whatever possibilities your spine is capable of.

Within Spine Mechanics, there are five fundamentals of movement: *elasticity*, *chest dropping*, *belly consciousness*, *bone softening*, and *levity*. Although they appear to work independently of each other, with experience they come together, working simultaneously, thereby becoming unified and second nature.

## ELASTICITY

The spine is one of many miracles of evolution, allowing humans stable and sustainable upright, bipedal movement. Our spines have adapted to absorb *compression* (the gravitational load/stress of weight bearing or minor axial impact) and to accommodate *elongation* (skeletal traction/strain through stretching—either passively, as in unsupported suspension from the limbs, or actively, using musculoskeletal effort to create extension). Both of these movements, which are responsible for a spine's *elasticity*, rely on two primary components:

- The strength, suppleness, and cushioning provided by the intervertebral discs

- The alternating system of convex and concave curvature of the vertebral column, supported by the corresponding activity and mobility in paraspinal/intercostal connective tissue, with the coordinated action and alignment of the skull and pelvis

In one way, you can think of the spine as a life-sized Slinky, the classic toy from the 1940s made from a simple coiled steel spring. Both the Slinky and your spine are designed to elongate and compress in the linear axis, although accommodating compression in the spine is a little more complex than what's found in the toy. Where the Slinky uses only its coils to resist the force of being pushed together, the function of the spine relies on a combination of intervertebral discs and alternating spinal curves (lordosis and kyphosis) to resist dynamic or static loads placed on it.

In their role as shock absorbers, the intervertebral discs of the spine act like cushions, accommodating minor vertebral movement and, in conjunction with the vertebral column, protect the nerves in and around the spinal cord. The connective tissue of each disc comprises an outer ring of fibrocartilage with a gel-like center that, due to limited vascular access, relies on intermittent bouts of gentle compression and elongation for stimulating the circulation of nutrients (blood, lymph, and cranial-sacral hydration).

For its role, the curvature of the spine acts like a big S-shaped spring, distributing stress and strain from more dynamic vertebral mobility. In isolation, the movement within a single curve (cervical, thoracic, lumbar, sacral, coccyx) has limits to its range of motion, especially in reverse curvature. Also, neither the Slinky nor the spine is well equipped to absorb uneven, nonaxial forces against any of its various parts in isolation, especially with continued repetitive motion or sudden impact trauma. What this means in simple language is that by design, the spine is amazing, but you shouldn't abuse it by regularly going on high-velocity roller coasters that jolt your body laterally (side to side). And like the Slinky, the spine's integrity and sustainability lie in honoring the beauty of its design as a complete, holistic system. Moving repetitively with a flat back, as is commonly taught in forward-folding yoga poses, is overrated and precarious, not only for the overall health of the spine but also for the pressure or stress it places on adjacent anatomical structures and nerve plexuses—namely, the occipital/atlas joint, brain stem, and cervical nerve roots at the top and the sacral-lumbar/sacroiliac joints and sciatic and vagus nerves at the bottom.

Are there other ways for the spine to move, especially for bending forward, backward, or sideways, where the focus is less on a spine's extension (flatness) and more on the spine's suppleness (curves)? We have only to look for guidance from our playful guru, the Slinky.

If you can, imagine a Slinky "walking" down a flight of stairs (or search "slow motion stair Slinky" on YouTube). Notice how its bending motion is an even, perpetual curling, with momentum sustained by gravity; also notice how the compression from bending stress on the low side of the spring is evenly distributed throughout the coil. Witnessing a Slinky in motion gives you clues for alternative types of bending in the spine that will be explained further in the third Practice Principle, Fundamentals of Flow, in chapter 16.

Compression, as previously mentioned, is a necessary part of a healthy spine and is present in all but a few yoga poses. When a spine bends forward, intervertebral discs are compressed on their anterior aspect, especially in the lumbar and cervical regions; when a spine bends backward, the posterior aspect of the disc is compressed, especially in the thoracic; when a spine bends sideways, compression occurs on the inferolateral (lower side) aspect of the disc; and when a spine rotates or twists, the discs are gently compressed, much like a wet dish towel you wring out and notice it gets shorter. What helps the spine absorb compression is the release of unnecessary muscular contraction in the back and the subtle role gravity plays at any moment for initiating spinal movement evenly.

For example, if you try to extend any part of the spine using imposed muscular force when bending forward, especially a part you know to be vulnerable or that causes you anxiety, additional contraction of paraspinal muscles occurs when the back flattens. This further decreases the space between the vertebrae, increasing the compressive forces and further stressing the discs in the area of bending. To avoid that, you must learn how to spread the natural compressive stresses of any pose over the full length of the spine, allowing the natural cushioning and shock absorption of a complete system of intervertebral discs to be shared.

The Slinky shows us how simple elongation can be: hold one end, release the other, and let gravity do the work (*passive* elongation); or place the Slinky on its side, hold each end, and pull apart (*active* elongation). The most efficient method to move the spine operates in identical ways, and the following two poses are excellent examples.

Passive elongation in the spine is easily found and articulated in Downward-Facing Dog (*Adho Mukha Svanasana*), as shown in figure 10. The shape of this pose lets you release the skull end of the spine to gravity; for the tailbone end of the spine, instead of pulling the tailbone up as is commonly taught, the work is to keep the tailbone still while softening deep into your pelvis. Anatomically, stabilizing the coccyx without mentally imposed muscular force in the abdominals (i.e., actively pulling the navel in) or the abductors, gluteals, and urogenital and anal sphincters (i.e., actively lifting the tailbone up) requires a strong release in the skeletal and smooth muscle systems of the pelvic floor and pubis. This invites the muscles of the legs to engage and lengthen, keeping the hip joints from collapsing. To fully release the thoracic area of the spine requires an equal surrender in the shoulder girdle, chest, and throat, which invites the muscles of the arms to engage and lengthen, preventing the shoulder joints from collapsing.

**TO EXPERIENCE *PASSIVE ELONGATION* IN DOWNWARD-FACING DOG,** start on your hands and knees, feet hip width apart, toes tucked forward. With straight arms, place your hands slightly wider than shoulder width apart, fingers gently spread, pointing forward. Consciously slow your breath, maintaining an even rhythm: three- to four-second inhale and three- to four-second exhale, with the sound of breathing soft and smooth. On an exhale, slowly lift your knees off the floor and walk your feet back a little, extending your legs *toward* straight until you meet resistance in your hamstrings. Drop your head and push back against the hands, arms fully extended, hips moving back toward the heels.

With each inhale, follow the fullness of your breath into the back-body, feeling (or visualizing) the skin spreading across the collarbones, shoulder blades, lower back, and into the pelvic floor. Simultaneously, feel the expansion of your breath lifting you slightly, as if you were coming out of the pose.

With each exhale, consciously soften the collarbones and tops of the lungs (or visualize them softening), feel the weight of your armpits and heart dropping, and simultaneously engage your arms. At the same time, soften the sphincter muscles, the diaphragm, and the skin below your navel; feel the weight of your hips dropping; and at the same time, engage your legs.

For each cycle of breath, allow the inhale to lift you slightly, spine rounding one vertebra at a time; on the exhale, release your shoulders and engage the arms, and release your hips and engage the legs. Simultaneously, release the back of your skull, the sphincter muscles, and the skin below your navel, feeling the waist lengthen and the navel move in passively. After three cycles of breath, release and come out of the pose on an inhale.

The functional beauty in the physical shape of Downward-Facing Dog is its play between effort and surrender, between engaging and

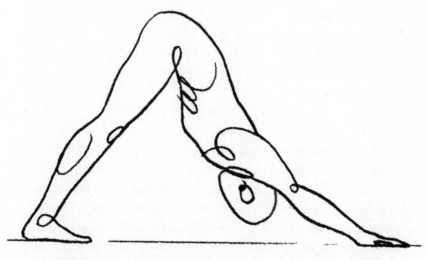

**FIGURE 10**   Downward-Facing Dog (*Adho Mukha Svanasana*)

releasing at the perimeter and core of the body simultaneously, as well as the attention and focus required to use your mind and your muscles together at multiple locations in the moment, all coordinated with your breathing.

For instance, by responding to gravity's downward pull on the heaviness found in your shoulders and hips as you release them, there is a natural response in the muscles of your arms and legs to engage as your nervous system becomes aware of the impending "danger" of collapsing and potential for collision with the floor. Additionally, a by-product of simultaneously releasing your shoulders while engaging your arms is passive external rotation of the upper-arm bone (humerus). This sets the shoulder and arm junction in an optimum position for support, strength, and flexibility. Likewise, by releasing the hips as you engage the legs, you create passive internal rotation of the upper-leg bone (femur), which optimally sets the hip and leg junction.

Also worth mentioning in this pose is the passive inward movement of the belly (*uddiyana bandha*) on the exhale as the diaphragmatic membrane releases its tension and returns up into the lower thoracic cavity. This action produces a vacuum effect (negative air pressure) in the abdominal cavity that draws the abdominal wall in slightly and supports the lengthening of the lower spine toward the tailbone. Experiencing this effortlessly in Downward-Facing Dog plants the seed for incorporating the practice of *bandhas* whenever you employ conscious breathing. To see a more detailed explanation and graphical representation of the subtle body components found in this pose, refer to "Subtle Body Guidesheet 3" in the appendix.

⁓

Active elongation in the spine is easily found and articulated in Mountain Pose (*Tadasana*), as shown in figure 11. The shape of this pose presents you with a simple exercise for tuning your balance, building poise, and increasing stability with minimal effort. Developing skill in basic poses like this proves useful as more challenging ones are introduced into your practice. The work in Mountain Pose is to release subconscious contraction in the front-body (i.e., collarbones, chest, and belly) and the musculature of the pelvic floor, while simultaneously engaging both ends of the spine in opposite directions (skull end actively up; coccyx end passively down).

Anatomically, to feel the pull of gravity passively on the coccyx without mentally imposed muscular effort (abdominals contracting the navel in; pelvic floor muscles pulling the tailbone down) requires a strong release in the diaphragm and the pubis in order to feel (or visualize) the weight of the abdominal organs settling into the pelvic floor. It simultaneously requires a strong release in the sphincter muscles (urogenital and anal), feeling the weight of the genitals sinking. The combination of these two downward gravitational "flows" from your torso produces a subtle feeling of heaviness through the perineum down into your legs and onto the feet, as well as deep awareness of connection to the ground beneath you. Grounding physically and energetically creates lightness, or *levity*, that instinctively elevates your body and your mood. When *levity* is felt, a blissful state appears with an enthusiastic urge to move further into your pose.

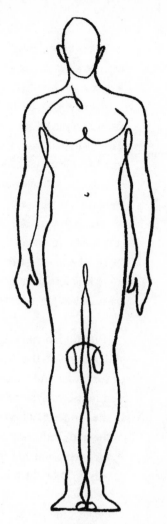

**FIGURE 11**
Mountain Pose (*Tadasana*)

**TO EXPERIENCE *ACTIVE ELONGATION* IN MOUNTAIN POSE,** start by standing upright with feet together, arms at your sides, palms facing each other, head upright. Consciously slow your breathing, with the sound of your breath soft, and the texture of your breath smooth. Slowly shift your weight back toward your heels without the toes lifting, until your thighs instinctively engage. Feel the subtle texture of your mat (or the floor) with your feet, the skin of your soles soft, toes passive. Soften your collarbones, feel the shoulders dropping, and gently extend your fingertips downward.

With each inhale, follow the fullness of your breath into the front, side, and back of the lungs, the full length of your torso. Feel (or visualize) the subtle expansion of the breath filling you.

With each exhale, consciously soften your diaphragm and feel the weight of your abdominal organs falling; release the collarbones, feel the shoulders sinking; soften the tops of the lungs, feel the heart dropping; and keep extending your fingertips. Simultaneously, draw the chin in (not down) slightly toward your throat, keeping the forehead still, and feel the back of the skull lifting naturally toward the crown; at the same time, release the sphincter muscles and feel (or visualize) the tailbone falling.

For each cycle of breath, allow the inhale to fill you—front, side, and back, into the pelvic floor; on the exhale, re-release your diaphragm, feel the abdominal organs dropping and resting on the pelvic floor; re-release the sphincter muscles and feel the tailbone and genitals sinking while keeping the spine engaged gently from the back of the skull, chin in slightly toward the throat. After five cycles of breath, release the pose and remain standing.

The functional beauty in the physical shape of Mountain Pose is its ability to reveal the dynamic qualities of stillness and balance, the power of surrender and intuitive response in the moment, and the coordination to use your mind and muscles simultaneously at multiple locations in the moment, all coordinated with your breath. As with all positions of the body requiring balance, adept and coordinated positioning of the head, torso, and lower limbs organized around your body's center of gravity helps reduce unnecessary muscular effort. Like the Slinky, the most efficient way to elongate the spine is to engage both of its ends while keeping the lumbar and thoracic spine passive—at the top by lifting the skull end of the spine up actively, while simultaneously releasing the tailbone end of the spine down passively.

To see a more detailed explanation and graphical representation of the subtle body components found in this pose, refer to "Subtle Body Guidesheet 2" in the appendix.

## CHEST DROPPING

As you gain more understanding of *elasticity* and experience the role its components of compression and elongation play in healthy movement, the importance of *chest dropping* grows, especially the lead it takes in releasing subconscious tension around the thoracic spine, which is necessary for effortless elongation. This span of vertebrae (T1–T12) has a more complex musculoskeletal arrangement than the rest, due to the attachment of twenty-four articulating ribs, intercostal muscles, and multiple bands of connective tissue that support movement in the floating bones of the shoulder—the scapulae (shoulder blades) and clavicles (collarbones) that secure the arms to the trunk.

The chest cavity (thorax) forms the upper part of the torso between the neck and the abdomen, formed by the rib cage (ribs, sternum, and spine) and associated connective tissue, which includes the diaphragm at the bottom of the rib cage. Within the thoracic cavity are the heart and lungs—chief organs of the cardiovascular and respiratory systems.

For decades, I trained as a "chest lifter," first working with weights in gyms and later during yoga practice. The action of lifting my chest was so ingrained that it became an involuntary position for the front of my body. I was unaware that even when I was in a relaxed state, a subconscious grip was maintaining the lift. As is true of many yoga classes today, I strongly emphasized chest lifting for reasons that now seem completely nonsensical. Here is a partial list of the yogic or spiritual justifications I used: opening the heart (physically and psychologically), better breathing and increased range, maximum spinal extension when forward bending to help maintain a neutral curve of the lumbar, and "protecting" the lower back by forcing the hips to fold. There are two other reasons I suspect for the popularity of lifting the chest—to overcome rounded shoulders (what keyboard junkies fear most) and to escape the social stigma that comes with being "flat chested."

To understand the effectiveness of *chest dropping*, let's look a little closer at two central misconceptions of chest lifting. First, to create "maximum spinal extension," in whole or in part, by lifting the chest, the paraspinal muscles of the thorax and the posterior intercostal muscles of the ribs engage. All muscle engagement creates a state of contraction, which ultimately causes a shortening or loss of extension (compression) in the spine. To overcome contraction caused by chest lifting, the thoracic muscles that engage when the chest lifts must be released. When the chest drops, these muscles are naturally passive, which allows the lower cervical and thoracic portions of the spine to move freely with the fundamental of elongation, where the ends of the spine—the tailbone and the back of the skull—are gently pulled apart, actively or passively. To free up the lumbar region of the spine, the diaphragm and skin below the navel must also release.

During the physical action of "opening the heart" by lifting the chest, the inner edges of the scapulae (shoulder blades) engage, pressing against the thoracic vertebrae—a very mobile part of the spine capable of reverse curvature in backbends. As the thoracic vertebrae are pressed and move forward, they, in turn, press into the back of your heart. With a relaxed spine, the heart gently rests against your sternum. However, when the chest lifts, your spine engages, and the resting heart gets trapped against your relatively immobile sternum, which acts like a keystone for your rib cage, connected by costal cartilages with limited mobility, since your thoracic spine has a far greater range of motion. Even if you attempt to lift the ribs and sternum to make space for the heart and a deeper breath, the intercostal muscles naturally contract when inhaling; thus, breathing deep with this form of lifting is not only counterproductive but also mostly ineffective for increasing the physical capacity of your lungs and heart. When the chest lifts, the heart is literally squeezed, putting strain on the cardiac muscle tissue, which limits the flow of blood into and out of the heart. In addition, the ribs contract, putting strain on the lungs' ability to breathe freely and access all five lobes (three in the right lung, two in the left).

Psychologically, opening the heart with chest lifting doesn't hold up well either. Think about this: We use the expression "openhearted" to describe those who are kind, generous, loving, and naturally inclined toward intimacy. I enjoy using the following metaphor, modeled by two student volunteers for effect, when introducing this idea in workshops:

> Imagine two people, say in a new relationship living
> in different countries, reuniting after an extended and
> lonely time apart. After a long journey to meet again,
> the moment has finally arrived. Standing in a terminal,

a flow of passengers streaming by, our lovers excitedly look to catch the first glimpse of their beloved. At last their eyes meet (are you getting the picture?), the anticipation peaking. They run toward each other (in slow motion, of course!), and right at the last moment before their luscious embrace, both chest lift to hug.

Absurd, right? Not even a remote possibility, unless it's two football players after a touchdown! To physically express the kind of emotion two lovers are feeling in that moment elicits a more receptive chest, soft and sensitive for meeting and receiving the other with the most contact two bodies could make. In other words, chest dropping, skin tingling, heart beating, electricity flowing, shoulders and breath naturally expanding, with arms gently enveloping the other, souls merging. Now imagine if that was your new experience every time you found yourself in a yoga pose involving *chest dropping*.

*Chest dropping* for bending forward is isolated and articulated in Seated Straight-Leg Forward Bend (*Paschimottanasana*), as shown in figure 12. In this variation of the classic pose, the hands are placed on the thighs to support the legs to accommodate full release of muscular effort, feeling the legs empty and simultaneously softening deep into the pelvic floor. If your hands don't reach the lower thighs, use a yoga strap to bind your legs

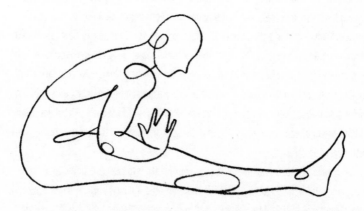

**FIGURE 12**   Seated Straight-Leg Forward Bend (*Paschimottanasana*)

in the same place, and rest your hands flat on the floor with straight arms to lean as far forward as gravity allows without anxiety.

As with Mountain Pose, the work in this pose is to release subconscious contraction in the front-body (i.e., collarbones, chest, and belly) and the musculature of the pelvic floor, while simultaneously engaging both ends of the spine in opposite directions (skull end actively up; coccyx end passively down). However, to create elongation in the spine and move deeper into this pose, which furthers hip and hamstring flexibility, the action of *chest dropping* triggers a stronger gravitational pull on the torso and provides the primary force to safely take you lower into the pose. Gravity-initiated movement is uniquely suited for everyone and produces the perfectly calibrated amount of weight or force to take you deeper. Anatomically, to fully feel the pull of gravity down on the chest requires a conscious softening into the top of the lungs as you exhale (this occurs naturally but is most often subconscious). As the tops of the lungs soften, the pericardium (the fibroserous sac of connective tissue filled with fluid that protects your heart) also softens, and you can feel the weight of your heart sinking energetically. As the heart sinks (or as you visualize it sinking), there is a sensation of "inner space" opening in what was formerly occupied by the now sinking heart, which gives you an opportunity for effortless slow breathing.

**TO EXPERIENCE *CHEST DROPPING* IN SEATED STRAIGHT-LEG FORWARD BEND,** sit with straight legs, feet together, toes pointing up. With your hands, pull the flesh of your buttocks away from the sitting bones (ischial tuberosities). Consciously slow your breathing, maintaining an even rhythm (three- to four-second inhale; three- to four-second exhale). Keep the sound of your breath soft and smooth. On an exhale, lean forward, placing the heels of your palms onto the sides of your thighs, just above the knees, fingers pointing up. Keep your head in line with your neck and slide the chin in slightly toward your throat without the forehead dropping, extending the back of your skull toward the crown, elbows gently pressing forward.

With each inhale, follow the fullness of your breath into the back-body, feeling (or visualizing) the skin spreading across the shoulder blades, lower back, and into the pelvic floor. Simultaneously, feel the expansion of your breath lift you slightly, as if you were coming out of the pose.

With each exhale, soften the collarbones and feel your armpits (shoulders) dropping, soften the tops of your lungs and feel your heart dropping, soften the diaphragm and feel your abdominal organs dropping, and soften the sphincter muscles (anal and urinary) and feel your genitals sinking. "Empty" your legs, gently pressing the knees together with your hands. Feel your tailbone dropping as you simultaneously draw the chin in slightly toward the throat, with the back of the skull moving up toward the crown.

For each cycle of breath, inhale through the back-body, coming out of the pose slightly, spine rounding. On the exhale, re-release through the front-body, with the chest, shoulders, and belly soft, organs dropping, legs passive; simultaneously engage the spine from the back of the skull, head in line with the neck, hands supporting the knees, as you gently press your elbows forward and allow gravity to take you lower. After five cycles of breath, release the pose and sit up with an inhale.

The functional beauty in the physical shape of Seated Straight-Leg Forward Bend is how such a simple pose can be so confronting, especially for students with tight hamstrings. Because of its intensity, this pose forces the mind to stay present in places where discomfort is greatest, which is perfect since this is where the most work is required. However, it has less to do with stretching and muscling your way further and more to do with softening and releasing yourself lower. Unlike in Downward-Facing Dog, gravity's influence for elongation of the spine is minimal, and its presence is felt more for muscular and joint releases in the legs, groin, and hips. This is where *chest dropping* becomes the hidden subtle body force that allows you to move safely and gently into your pain, at your own pace; it also gives you opportunities to uncover how to respond to intensity, both physically (releasing contraction) and mentally (reducing anxiety).

To see a more detailed explanation and graphical representation of the subtle body components found in this pose, refer to "Subtle Body Guidesheet 5" in the appendix.

*Chest dropping* for bending backward is isolated and articulated in Standing Backbend (*Utthita Dhanurasana*), as shown in figure 13. This is another variation of a classic pose, where the hands are placed behind

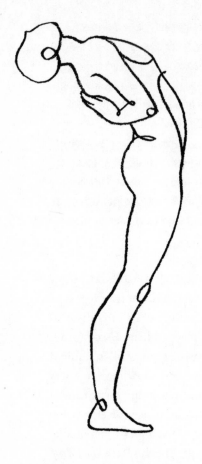

**FIGURE 13** Standing Backbend
(*Utthita Dhanurasana*)

your back, palms together, fingers pointing up, to allow your forearms to support the lower back ribs and your hands to support your upper thoracic vertebrae. If your shoulders or wrists are stiff, be creative with modifications. (If needed, with your hands behind your back, bring the tops of your wrists together, fingers pointing down; or even easier, just grab your elbows behind your back.) To create more support for your lower back, the elbows are gently pressed forward (not back), which forms a shelf on which to rest your kidneys and floating ribs. If there are limitations in your neck, find an adjustable harness that you can hang from a ceiling or wall to support your head, or simply practice this pose next to a tall bookcase that's securely anchored to a wall and let your head rest on an empty shelf, perhaps using small cushions on the shelf to be comfortable or to fine-tune the height. Whenever you're using props, be sure they're strong and steady. If you feel any anxiety using them, correct that before proceeding.

In this pose, the action of *chest dropping* is similar to Seated Straight-Leg Forward Bend, except the spine bends in the opposite direction. Dropping through the chest in this pose relies on the fundamental of spinal *elasticity* and its ability to spread back-bending stresses evenly over the entire length of the vertebral column. As with the Slinky, the field of gravity that operates evenly on the spine when surrender is present is the only force necessary to bend backward. It works best when you're able to fully release tension in the front-body (collarbones, throat, top of the lungs, and diaphragm) and feel the weight of your internal organs sinking toward the back-body. This action will release the unnecessary tension in your back and let the necessary tension—the naturally occurring tension in response to the give and take when balancing—remain. It's not something you have to think about, as long as your body maintains its center of gravity and the spine stays engaged lightly from the ends (tailbone sinking; back of skull extending).

At first when practicing this way in backbends—especially if your only experience so far has been with chest lifting—you can create support for the vulnerable parts of the spine by gently pressing the elbows and outer shoulders forward, which supports the spine in two ways: it engages your trapezius muscles, which lift slightly and create a trapeze-like cradle for the neck; and it drives your forearms forward, creating a similar support for the lumbar spine, as well as the kidneys and floating ribs. This pose demands trust in the strength of your spine; initially, if you lack that trust, your range of motion should be minimal. Do only what you can do without anxiety and save the rest for another day.

TO EXPERIENCE *CHEST DROPPING* IN STANDING BACKBEND, stand with your feet hip width apart, feet parallel, arms at your sides. Consciously slow your breathing, with the sound of your breath soft, and the texture of your breath smooth. Feel the subtle texture of your mat (or the floor) with your feet, the skin of your soles soft, toes passive. When ready, on an inhale, lift the arms out to the sides, shoulder height, and then internally rotate your arms as you sweep them behind you, bringing the palms together behind your back with fingers pointing up. (Use the variations noted above if needed.) As you exhale, release your collarbones, feel your shoulders drop a little, and gently press your elbows and outer shoulders forward, forearms firm against the back ribs, hands firm against the thoracic spine. Slowly lean your hips forward without the heels lifting, keeping the belly and butt soft, legs firm. Draw your chin in slightly toward the throat as you take the head back and look up, neck resting in the trapeziums.

With each inhale, follow (visualize) your breath into the back of the heart, feel the skin spread across your shoulder blades; breathe into the kidneys, feel the skin spread across the floating ribs; and breathe into the rectum, feeling its subtle expansion press into the sacroiliac joints and down into the pelvic floor. Allow the fullness of your breath to lift you slightly out of the pose.

With each exhale, re-release your collarbones, feel your shoulders fall away from the ears; press the hips, elbows, and outer shoulders gently forward, while simultaneously softening the tops of the lungs; feel your heart sinking. Soften the diaphragm, releasing the weight of your abdominal organs down into the pelvic floor; soften the lower back ribs (see "Bone Softening," later in this chapter) as they meet and rest on your forearms and hands. Simultaneously extend the spine through the back of the skull, with the thoracic spine resting on the hands, chin sinking in slightly toward the throat, neck supported by the trapeziums, with your head at rest.

With each cycle of breath, inhale through the back-body, feeling the breath lift you slightly, expanding the skin across your back the full length of your torso. On the exhale, consciously soften the front-body and feel the weight of your internal organs falling, resting on the spine; gently press the hips forward, belly and butt soft, legs strong, feeling the texture of your mat with your feet. As gravity takes you deeper, gaze toward the ceiling or the wall behind you. After three cycles of breath, inhale coming up, head last; release your hands, dropping the arms to your sides. Remain standing in Mountain Pose and feel the subtle body effects of this pose.

The functional beauty in the physical shape of Standing Backbend is how enjoyable and effortless bending backward can be when gravity is the final authority for how deeply you enter the pose. Be patient and allow the spine to unfold—don't push. For many, bending backward is difficult and sometimes frightening at first; yet, to maintain balance in a healthy spine, backbends are a primary, sustaining force. Generally we function in a forward-facing, right-side-up world, relying heavily on our eyes for our sense of identity and direction. We orientate our position in the world, both personally and spatially, through our eyes. Because our sense of position is often a function of seeing, in many backbends, we lose our habitual way of relating to our environment and must learn to cultivate another sense for seeing (and positioning). The shape of this pose places your head back and vision above or behind the body, where your physical eyes lose their ordinary frame of reference. It can be an alien experience as your "worldview" is literally turned upside down. Your normal context for relating to yourself (and the image that sustains you) becomes lost.

With the fear that comes from this loss of context, there is a common reaction where your breathing becomes short or your breath is held. In addition, there is often a habitual contraction in the muscles of your buttocks and abdomen, and the neck, if weak, becomes vulnerable as the shoulders grip for protection. When these reactions are present in your body, the movement in this pose does not respond well to overloading, or excessive muscular force. The pose feels out of balance, and the more you struggle, the less the pose responds. This only deepens the frustration, and you are likely to give up or check out. If this happens, back out of the pose a little and reestablish a slow rhythm to your breathing. Follow the sensation of your breath in and out of the areas where resistance or gripping resides. See if this type of breathing reduces the anxiety. If not, slowly exit the pose altogether, returning to it again the next time you practice.

To see a more detailed explanation and graphical representation of the subtle body components found in this pose, refer to "Subtle Body Guidesheet 4" in the appendix.

## BELLY CONSCIOUSNESS

For optimum forward, back, and side bending or for twisting in the waist and lumbar region of the spine, the abdominal muscles and internal organs must be free of unnecessary tension. Like *chest dropping* in backbends, the fundamental of *belly consciousness* is an idea that contradicts most of the yoga technique and theory currently in vogue. As we saw in part 3, the belly region of the body is not a simple thing, nor is it one that is easily integrated when we begin our yoga practice with a "bellyful" of conditioning and habitual behavior. The challenge here is to learn (or relearn) how to move, even when stiffness is present, with a minimum of muscular effort—how to turn or bend from where genuine movement is anchored, free of mental imposition or rote technique.

The belly holds many keys for maintaining balance, as well as an unshakable connection to our center of gravity physically and our seat of intuition psychically. When every movement we make in yoga springs from the belly, it produces a smooth, effortless motion rooted in the center of ourselves, with full presence of mind and the stamina we truly possess. The diaphragm, the navel, and the space just below the navel are powerful areas for releasing tension, especially that which is subconscious and located elsewhere. As we learned in part 4, the subtle energy center located below the navel (*svadhisthana*) is the seat of our water element—literally, the trigger for fluidity—in our bodies. By releasing tension in the belly and using a slow, conscious breath, we activate the vagus nerve, which is the gateway into the parasympathetic nervous system, the master controller for releasing tension throughout the body. With mental focus placed in other areas where tension is present, releasing the belly facilitates targeted relaxation elsewhere.

*Belly consciousness* is isolated and articulated in Seated Crossed-Leg Twist (*Parivrtta Sukhasana*), as shown in figure 14. In this pose, the arms are used for leverage to turn the waist on the exhale cycle of the breath, as the diaphragm releases and the weight of the abdominal organs drops, creating more space to twist from. The front-body is passive, and the spine stays engaged gently from the back of the skull. Each inhalation cycle allows the spine to unwind a little, as the expansion of your breath takes you slightly out of the pose. Each exhalation cycle creates a deeper release in the belly, a gentle softening in the top of the lungs (*chest dropping*) and, using the arms for leverage, a simultaneous rotation in the waist and elongation of the spine by extending the back of the skull. Dropping the opposite shoulder to the knee on an exhale completes the pose.

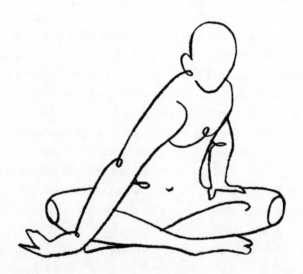

**FIGURE 14** Seated Crossed-Leg Twist (*Parivrtta Sukhasana*)

Anatomically, twisting through the waist tones our gastric metabolism by boosting circulation of blood and lymph, which ultimately strengthens the digestive organs (liver, gall bladder, and pancreas), which secrete enzymes, hormones, and bile to break down and transmute the food we eat. The process of transmuting food on the physical level is supported in your subtle body by one of the five processes (*pancha vayus*) known as *samana* ("that which balances or pacifies"), located at the navel and responsible for regulating one of the five elements (*pancha bhutas*) known as *agni* ("fire"). Exercises of the waist, including twists and bending (forward, back, and side), also help provide relief for minor back spasms, reduce stiffness in the hips, and release chronic tension in the diaphragm. Working with this pose also increases your awareness and presence of your true center and helps purify the body from the core (*hara*), physically and psychologically.

TO EXPERIENCE *BELLY CONSCIOUSNESS* IN SEATED CROSSED-LEG TWIST, start by sitting with legs crossed, your knees lined up over your feet and shinbones parallel. With your hands, pull the flesh of your buttocks away from the sitting bones (ischial tuberosities). Consciously slow your breathing, maintaining an even rhythm (three- to four-second inhale and three- to four-second exhale). Keep the sound of your breath soft and smooth. Take your right hand around the front of the right knee and turn the top of your wrist down into the floor, fingers pointing out to the side, elbow straight. Place the left hand at the head of the thigh, near the hip crease, palm pressing down and fingers pointing forward. Inhale slowly, following the sensation of your breath through the back into the pelvic floor, with the torso unwinding slightly (out of the pose). On the exhale, using your arms for leverage, press your right shoulder forward, pull the left shoulder back, and twist through your waist, keeping the belly soft, organs dropping, chest dropping. Keep your head in line with your neck, chin in line with your sternum, torso leaning forward slightly.

With each inhale, come out of the pose slightly (unwinding), feeling the fullness of your breath through the back into the pelvic floor.

With each exhale, soften your diaphragm, feel the abdominal organs dropping, navel receding slightly, top of the lungs softening, heart dropping; simultaneously turn through the shoulders and the waist, keeping the spine engaged from the back of the skull.

After two to three cycles of breath, inhale fully. Then exhale until you're empty. Holding the breath out, slowly lower the right shoulder to the left knee, keeping the right arm straight. Stay down, holding your breath out for as long as you can without anxiety. When you need to, slowly inhale and come up, unwinding out of the pose. Change arms and repeat on the second side.

The functional beauty in the physical shape of Seated Crossed-Leg Twist is how enjoyable and effortless twisting can be when surrender in the belly and chest determines how deeply you enter the pose. Without "muscling" your twists, be patient and allow the spine to spiral/twist naturally with each release of your exhale, feeling the fluidity that comes with softness, which takes pressure off the diaphragm and naturally invites you to twist deeper.

To see a more detailed explanation and graphical representation of the subtle body components found in this pose, refer to "Subtle Body Guidesheet 7" in the appendix.

## BONE SOFTENING

At a very early point in life, your bones were naturally capable of bending for what was absolutely necessary to survive your first "journey," out of the womb and through the birth canal. Physically and energetically, this memory still exists in your DNA and nervous system.

Borrowing from *chi kung's* martial art practice of Bone Marrow Washing, the fundamental of *bone softening* allows you to feel deeply into yourself—a forgotten art that survives only as an expression of intuition in English: "I feel it in my bones." As you rediscover the sensitivity to feel into your bones, it becomes a useful skill to channel gravity's effect as a subtle force for skeletal movement when all other means to move are inaccessible, too intense, or too crude. This is especially true when working with soft tissue injuries or joint mobility limitations.

Feeling softness in your bones starts with visualization by placing your attention where softness still exists physically: the gelatinous, spongy marrow found in the core of your bones. To feel with this level of sensitivity takes time and patience, so keep visualizing until the feeling comes to you.

*Bone softening* and its effect on your ability to move when experiencing intense sensation are found in the simple yet challenging Standing Side Bend (*Akarasana*), shown in figure 15. The shape of this pose naturally creates a confrontation with stiffness in the waist through a strong lateral stretch on the upside of your torso, from the hip through the upper waist, ribs, shoulder, and arm. On the downside, your torso is put into acute compression, often creating intensity so strong that it can literally take your breath away. Another useful effect of this pose is the temporary distortion it creates between each lung—as the lower rib cage and waist are compressed, the lower lung is restricted; as the upper rib cage and waist are lengthened, the upper lung is expanded.

Psychologically, this pose may cause anxiety when inhaling, until you learn "bipolar" breathing (isolating breath into each lung separately). Anatomically, what feels like bone (your floating ribs) meeting bone (your iliac crest) is more accurately the connective tissue that joins the bony upper and lower boundaries of your waist being deeply squeezed as the lower waist compresses. To move deeper into this pose, *bone softening* is used to free up the physical and psychological grip produced by anxiety; this anxiety naturally appears when the side-bending shape approaches the edge of your strength or flexibility, in the intercostal muscles of the lower rib cage and the connective tissues of the waist.

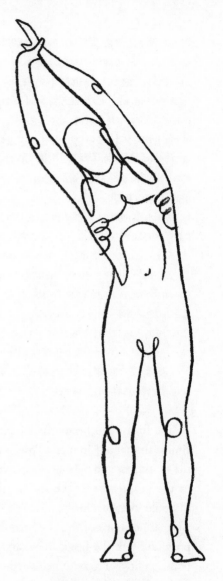

**FIGURE 15** Standing Side Bend (*Akarasana*)

**TO EXPERIENCE *BONE SOFTENING* IN STANDING SIDE BEND,** place your feet parallel, hip width apart. On an inhale, take your arms overhead, and with your right hand, grab the left wrist and pull the left arm straight beside (or behind) your head. Shift your weight onto the right foot and, with an exhale, side bend to the right. Feel the texture of your mat (or the ground) with your feet, keeping the toes passive. Keep your breathing slow, with the sound of your breath soft and smooth. At every step of the way, you can control the intensity of the pose by how much you lean into it; let your breath be your guide. If your breathing is labored, back out of the pose a little and regain control over the sound (soft and smooth) and rhythm (slow) of your breath.

With each inhale, feel the fullness of your breath into the upper lungs and back-body, lifting you slightly out of the pose. Where physical intensity is present, "touch" its discomfort as softly as you can with the cool, subtle expansion produced by your breath.

With each exhale, consciously soften the lower ribs and diaphragm, feeling gravity gently pulling down on your abdominal organs as the diaphragm releases and the torso sinks deeper into the pose. Notice how the amount of extension you create in the arms overhead gives you control over how much intensity you allow and increases the leverage gravity provides for a passive opportunity for *bone softening* in the lower ribs to take you deeper into the pose.

After three cycles of breath, come out of the pose on an inhale, switch arms, shift your weight to the other side, and repeat.

The functional beauty in the physical shape of Standing Side Bend, similar to that of Mountain Pose, is its ability to reveal the dynamic qualities of stillness and balance, the power of surrender and intuitive response in the moment, and the use of mind and muscles simultaneously at multiple locations in the moment, all coordinated with your breath. As with all positions of the body requiring balance, adept and coordinated positioning of the head, torso, and lower limbs organized around your body's center of gravity helps reduce unnecessary muscular effort. The understanding gained through using *bone softening* in this pose can be applied to any pose where bony parts of your body meet hard surfaces or each other, providing you with a means to meet any experience of intensity with presence and poise, trusting that your body and mind working together will uncover the appropriate response to move deeper.

To see a more detailed explanation and graphical representation of the subtle body components found in this pose, refer to "Subtle Body Guidesheet 6" in the appendix.

## LEVITY

The last and most essential fundamental of Spine Mechanics is *levity*. As we discussed in chapter 4, *levity* is a by-product of gravity, which is a foundational basis of Newtonian physics. But it was something early yogis uncovered long before Newton's "discoveries."

When our upright bodies experience the downward pull of gravity in a yoga pose, a hidden force exists that we rely on to resist it. Through understanding and applying *levity*, we learn to activate it in our physical body and use this force that gravity naturally provides. We can also feel its influence on our subtle body and its effects on our psychology, which is literally a layer of our body that is the seat of our feelings and emotions (*manomaya kosha*). It is here that *levity*, or "lightness of heart," produces a psychological effect that naturally influences our endocrine glands (feel-good hormones) and nervous system (parasympathetic response), which in turn help provide ease in movement and in life. When we manifest this type of *levity*, we see our world more clearly, feel our relationships more authentically, and learn more about ourselves through intimate connection to others and the natural world within and outside of ourselves.

Ultimately, when we fully integrate the fundamental of *levity*, our life becomes a natural expression of deep gratitude for the mindful, breath-full movement it produces. This body-mind process reawakens wonder, inspiration, and delight, which support us at any stage of life. It helps us avoid taking yoga or ourselves too seriously and reveals a more intuitive approach to living in the most refreshing and enlightening ways.

*Levity* provides guidance for movement with simple, sustainable, and efficient means. Paradoxically, it is initiated through the absence of physical effort—through surrender. It starts by realizing the potential in our relationship to the ground beneath us, which is where whatever part of our body meets the surface we are on. When that relationship is firmly established through intimacy (as with any good relationship, right?), we can anticipate with hyper-alertness how the subtle effects of gravity, coupled with surrender, can produce grace—a subtle opening that happens when surrender is present. In that moment, movement is initiated with nonmuscular effort, as our musculature intuitively responds to the subtle opening. This provides clues for more movement further into a pose.

This is a radically different approach from movement generated by mentally imposed muscular effort.

Inversions are perfect poses for mastering this fundamental, and I will use one of the most important poses in *hatha* yoga—Headstand—to demonstrate the process.

According to B. K. S. Iyengar, regular practice of Headstand "provides health and vitality for the brain, the master regulator of the sense organs and the seat of the soul (Brahman)" and is considered the Father (or King) of all yoga poses.[107]

Those new to inversions and those working with a preexisting condition in the spine (especially the neck or lower back), in the eyes (especially glaucoma or detached retina), or in the circulatory system (especially hypo/hypertension, blood clots, or stroke) should take extreme care when practicing this pose and bring more acute attention and slower movements to any inverted position to avoid strain from overuse, serious injury, or reinjury of an existing ailment. Any doubt you may have is a sign you should do these poses *only* under the guidance of a qualified instructor. For women, it is also recommended in the lifestyle wellness practices of *Ayurveda* to avoid the practice of inversions during menstruation.

If guidance from a teacher is not possible, spend several weeks working daily with a variety of asymmetrical standing poses (e.g., Triangle Pose, Lateral Angle Pose, Half-Moon Pose) to build strength and tone in the neck; Bridge Pose and Shoulderstand to help reduce stiffness in the neck; and Downward-Facing Dog, forearm balancing poses, and handstands at the wall to educate the arms, torso, and abdomen in how to soften and support alignment in the spine when upside down.

Experiencing the powerful effect *levity* promises can be isolated and articulated in the Headstand (*Sirsasana*) sequence, shown in figure 16. In this two-step pose, the alignment of the torso and legs precisely over the head into an anatomically neutral position holds the key for releasing unnecessary muscular force, especially in the arms and shoulders. The prerequisite effort to lift into the pose with one leg leading (step 1) helps prevent a premature launch that might lack the necessary core strength or spinal stability to protect the neck when both legs are elevated (step 2). The work of the arms is the same for both, providing only what is necessary for checking your balance to remain stable laterally and helping to keep your collarbones engaged and lifting away from the floor, which offers protection from minor instability or weakness of the cervical vertebral column (neck).

To experience *levity* in Headstand requires elongation at both ends of the spine, not by lifting but by trusting your spine's natural capacity to support either upright or inverted postures with minimal effort.

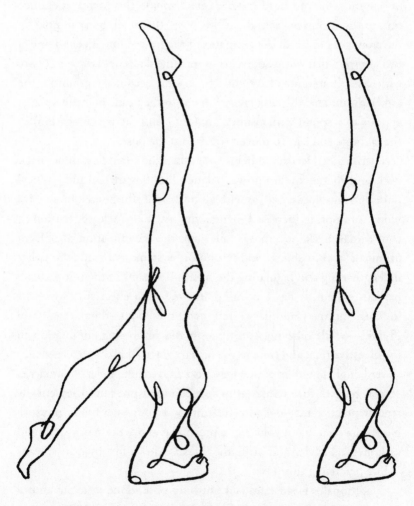

**FIGURE 16**  Headstand variations (*Sirsasana*, steps 1 and 2)

It is much like an inverted Mountain Pose; as long as the anatomical integrity (curvature) of your spine is maintained and your spatial sensitivity is finely tuned to the sensation of gravity moving through you and guiding your instinctive reflex when surrender is present, physical lightness (*levity*) in the spine is a natural by-product, and the musculature of your body responds intuitively to move you into a more stable pose. Specifically, as you exhale with a conscious softening of the diaphragm and tops of the lungs, the gravitational pull on your thoracic and abdominal organs creates a downward subtle body flow of sensation to your head (*passive compression*). This increases connection to the "primary ground" in this pose (the small, bony dimple on the crown of our head, the remnants of the frontal fontanel and one of two soft spots that we possessed in our infantile skulls until the age of two) with a small amount of weight left on our "secondary ground" (the arms). Simultaneously, as gravity is felt into the head, an intuitive urge appears to respond with a subtle amount of lift (active elongation) in the tailbone and legs to move further into the pose.

Specifically, Headstand helps strengthen the shoulders, upper back, neck, and abdomen. It improves balance, building mental and physical poise and steadiness, and, as with all inversions, flushes the brain with blood, promoting increased mental vitality. It also releases tension in your throat, neck, and thorax; alleviates the accumulation of phlegm or mucus in your sinuses and respiratory system; and gradually assists in lengthening and regulating the breath. In terms of the sympathetic nervous system, it has a calming and restoring effect. It also assists in balancing the glandular secretions in the body—the adrenals and thyroid—while relieving constipation and improving elimination in the digestive tract and tone in the urinary tract. Those with a tendency toward high blood pressure may also find relief. Inversions trigger several reflexes that temporarily reduce blood pressure; theoretically, regular practice may enhance treatment of your high blood pressure. Note, however, that if your blood pressure is above normal, you should seek medical advice and bring the pressure down first by other means before practicing this pose.

Traditionally Headstand is a finishing pose, done near the end of your practice session, either before Shoulderstand, which is known as a neck counterpose for Headstand, or after Shoulderstand, which is used as a neck opener and toner for Headstand. In either case, consistent and patient presence is recommended to gain mastery over Headstand to prepare you for relaxation, *pranayama*, and meditation.

As a transition from a practice based on movement, the finishing poses are practices based on stillness; they tap into the natural process of relaxation and healing in the body by helping pacify the nerves, soothe the brain and heart, and regulate the breath. This helps develop the calm alertness necessary for *pranayama*. When your practice of yoga *asana* and *pranayama* is consistent and thorough, deeper levels of meditation are possible, and the natural healing and immune response in your body gains strength, physically and psychologically.

Although there are many different approaches to the practice of Headstand, there can sometimes be confusion for beginners whether to "lift" or "hop" up; with straight or bent legs; with one leg or two; with arms bent, forearms on the floor, fingers interlocked, and hands cupping the back of the skull or with arms bent, forearms vertical, palms flat, and hands shoulder width apart in tripod. Ultimately, the choice is yours, and so are its consequences. Your choice should guide you to understanding the reasons for your practice of Headstand, not because someone else said it's "good for you," but because you have discovered in its practice a truth that was meant for you to discover and that provides you with an inner self-authority to know which approach is best in this moment.

TO EXPERIENCE *LEVITY* IN HEADSTAND, start on your hands and knees, clear from any objects on the floor or obstacles overhead (close proximity to a wall is recommended for beginners). Lower onto your elbows, shoulder width apart, and interlock your fingers with your palms apart. Walk your knees forward a little; pull the navel in, rounding your spine, and slowly lower the crown of your head flat to the floor, hands cupping the back of the skull lightly. Press down into the forearms and lift the collarbones up, away from the floor.

STEP 1. Take one to two cycles of breath here, feeling the floor (or your mat) on the top of your skull, directly on the "primary ground," or fontanel. If the rhythm of your breath distorts, that means anxiety is present, so either restore the slow, even rhythm to your breath or come out and try it again another day. If you're ready, tuck your toes forward and slowly straighten your legs, lifting the hips and walking your feet forward until the outer hips are over (or nearly over) your shoulders. Keep lifting the collarbones strongly to support the thorax and prevent excessive curvature in the thoracic spine (hyperkyphosis); feel the weight of your upper body descending onto the crown of your head, adjusting the position of your head intuitively to avoid neck strain. Keep your breathing soft, slow, and smooth. If your balance is steady, point your feet and roll onto the tips of your big toes. Then lift one leg as high as you can, with your toes pointed, and feel the toes reaching upward, knee straight. As you continue lifting strongly through the (upper) leg, visualize your big toe touching the ceiling and notice how light your other foot feels on the floor, balancing on the tip of the big toe. Keeping the collarbones engaged, actively pull your navel in a little as you lift the upper leg even higher, creating a standing split position with your legs. *Don't* hop up. This part of the pose tones the abdominal muscles and builds the strength and flexibility in the legs and groin necessary for the full pose. Keep both legs extending, upper big toe reaching for the ceiling, lower big toe firmly pointing into the floor, until the power of the upper leg extending gently elevates (pulls) the lower foot off the floor a few inches. Pause here for one to two cycles of breath, "free balancing" in Headstand with a floating split position for the legs. Keep your collarbones lifting away from the floor, balancing evenly on the crown of the head, and notice the first wave of lightness appearing in your forearms, then the legs, and eventually the spine.

STEP 2. If your balance is steady "floating" and you feel ready for the next step, keep both legs straight and slowly move the upper leg back a little farther, letting the lower leg lift passively while maintaining perfect equilibrium between your legs. Continue to let the upper leg drop back farther and feel the lower leg being pulled slowly up in front until your legs are level in a fully inverted forward-split position of the legs in Headstand. If this is your first time free balancing and you feel like you've had enough, or if your neck is getting tired, slowly come down with the front leg first, the back leg naturally following until both feet are on the floor. Then bend your knees and come down into a common variation of Child's Pose—knees wide, hip width apart; arms extending forward, palms down, shoulder width apart, forehead flat on the ground; and rest in this pose, one of the simplest counterposes for Headstand.

However, if your balance, coordination, and strength in Headstand are still sustainable, actively pull the navel in slightly as you slowly "scissor" your legs together evenly until your feet touch, side by side, both legs vertical. Breathe slowly, especially if you're a little wobbly, and keep readjusting the collarbones up away from the floor, re-releasing any hardness or excessive grip of the interlocked fingers to keep the hands receptive and soft. With each exhale, re-release the diaphragm and skin below the navel and feel your abdominal organs sinking toward your chest, with the navel passively moving in toward the spine. As the navel moves in, actively draw it in a little more while simultaneously drawing the tailbone forward slightly (toward the genitals) and pulling the legs back a little (behind you). Think of these actions like squeezing a tube of toothpaste. As your hand squeezes the tube toward its core, the intercavity pressure increases, and the paste oozes out the end of the tube. It's an apropos example of how your spine responds to efforts you apply in Headstand in response to *levity*, which supports *elongation* in the spine.

Initially, you may keep your weight evenly distributed between the arms and the head, until your confidence increases and the wobbliness disappears. With consistent practice, you can begin to shift more of your weight onto the crown, with less effort in the arms, without dropping the collarbones. This requires more sensitivity in maintaining your body's center of gravity and your openness to grace and in discovering profound lightness of being (*levity*). With intuitive alignment, this sensation of lightness is felt all the way to the feet, and the heels actively extend to take the pose even higher.

After four to six cycles of breath, slowly lower the second leg on an inhale, followed by the first leg, while keeping the knees straight; lightly touch the toes to the floor. When both feet are down, drop the knees to the floor, sit back, and fold forward into Child's Pose, arms forward, palms flat, resting.

If you are working with the common limitations in the curvature of the neck—cervical hypolordosis (reverse curvature) or cervical hyperlordosis (exaggerated curvature)—explore slight variations to the position of your head and their effects on relieving strain or feelings of weakness in your neck. For instance, positioning your inverted body above the head so the weight of the pose lands more toward the frontal (anterior) rim of the fontanel, with slow, consistent practice, can be very helpful in restoring balanced curvature to a neck that has a minor or moderate imbalance of reverse curvature. Likewise, if you position your body above so the weight of the pose lands more toward the dorsal (posterior) rim of the fontanel, with equal effort and commitment, this can be very beneficial in restoring a balanced curvature to a neck that has a minor or moderate imbalance of exaggerated curvature.

As the experience of *levity* becomes more familiar, the intuitive response or signal to go further informs appropriate muscular effort to maintain balance and equilibrium. Challenging poses like Headstand become like child's play, full of innocence, curiosity, and self-discovery.

Learning to move in Headstand without excessive muscular force will develop the intelligence necessary for safe practice at any stage in life, where the lightness (*levity*) that lifts the spine and creates its suppleness is understood. With experience, practicing this pose regularly produces an increased level of vitality and health within the spine and all of the body's biological systems and metabolic processes.

To see a more detailed explanation and graphical representation of the subtle body components found in this pose, refer to "Subtle Body Guidesheet 8" in the appendix.

One of the most universal and distinctive features of optimal [flow] experience [is] people become so involved in what they are doing that the activity becomes spontaneous, almost automatic; they stop being aware of themselves as separate from the actions they are performing.

**Mihaly Csikszentmihalyi**

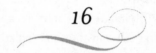

# *Fundamentals of Flow*

In the practice of *hatha* yoga, all movement becomes inseparable from conscious breathing, which supplies a deeper context for moving efficiently and forms an essential part of the third and final Practice Principle: Fundamentals of Flow. In *hatha* yoga, the word for "flow" is *vinyasa* and comes from two Sanskrit roots: *vi*, which denotes "in a special way," and *nyasa*, meaning "to place." The Fundamentals of Flow will help you place your attention in special ways to create present-moment awareness on three distinct levels of flow:

- **LEVEL 1:** Movement within a pose, linked with the rhythm and phases of the breath

- **LEVEL 2:** Movement in a sequence of poses, linked with smooth, graceful transitions between each pose

- **LEVEL 3:** Movement of one breath to the next, using slow, uninterrupted cycles linked seamlessly into one continuous stream of breathing

# LEVEL 1

Where body movement in a pose is linked with breathing, entering a pose is initiated with an exhale, and exiting a pose is initiated with an inhale (with very few exceptions). As you experience a pose, each inhale creates a momentary pause in movement, where the physical and subtle breath expand into the back-body or into a specific part of the body where resistance is present, or both. This creates a subtle sensation of buoyancy as you come out of the pose slightly (see "Inhalation (*Puraka*)" in chapter 14), while also producing a calming effect, giving you time to gather yourself and recognize any anxiety or subconscious grip you may be holding in a pose. With inhalation complete, a momentary retention of breath leads into a smooth transition to exhalation.

Each exhale while in a pose is a "call to action"; it is the moment when you release one or more areas in your body that chronically hold subconscious tension, mostly of a psychological nature. These areas can typically be found in the pelvic floor, the genitals, the skin below your navel, the diaphragm, the top of the lungs, the throat, the collarbones, the space between your eyebrows, and the scalp. Or you may simply gain an awareness of the "inner space" your subtle body provides anywhere you release resistance or discomfort in a pose. This creates a response in your parasympathetic nervous system, which in turn produces a sense of surrender and ease, and an intuitive invitation to move deeper into the space created by the exhale (see "Exhalation (*Rechaka*)" in chapter 14).

The process of softening generally occurs in the musculature of our front-body, in and around our internal organs, and/or in a specific area of the body where imbalance is conscious; it gradually releases physical and psychological resistance and allows gravity and intuitive response to move the body deeper into the pose until the end of the exhale. This continues with smooth transitions between each cycle of breath until the time in the pose is complete, typically one to three cycles of breath.

# LEVEL 2

When linking a sequence of poses, the importance of where you place your attention *when transitioning between* poses is equal to the importance of your attention *when being in* each pose. When this is achieved seamlessly, the choreography of your practice gives you the experience of one very long pose with a creative mix of variations, producing an unbroken stream of present-moment consciousness over an extended period. Creating a sequence that physically flows together *without* excessive amounts of repetitive "link" poses—think Downward-Facing Dog, Plank, Upward-Facing Dog, Plank, Downward-Facing Dog, and on to the next pose, repeated over and over again—requires a thorough understanding of the exit of each pose as its moving shape matches the entrance into each successive pose, with the minimum amount of effort required for a graceful transition. This also saves physical energy, as it conserves and strengthens life force and vital breath. This type of flow is used in the dynamic sequence (see "Practice Choreography" later in this chapter) and is generally vigorous, with heat-building poses held for short durations (usually one cycle of breath), producing strong effects in the cardiovascular and respiratory circulation of the body.

## LEVEL 3

In this level of linking uninterrupted cycles of the breath, where you place your attention affects both the physical and the subtle breath as a process of strengthening mental focus on the relatively simple task of conscious breathing. This type of *vinyasa* is the linking of one breath to the next, where breathing is experienced as if it were one long, continuous, flowing breath. This type of flow uses concentration on the three phases of breath—inhalation, exhalation, and retention (see "Phases of Breathing" in chapter 14)—and employs control of the three qualities of breath—sound, rhythm, and texture (see "Qualities of Breath" in chapter 14). Each of the three practice sequences (see "Basic Structure of Practice Sequences" later in this chapter) uses *breath-flow*, although in the opening and closing sequences, the rhythm quality of breath is likely to be slower than in the dynamic sequence.

## CREATING FLOW EFFORTLESSLY

Mastering the basics found in the Fundamentals of Flow helps reduce excessive repetition of individual poses or transitions, which tend to weaken the mind's ability to concentrate, resulting in boredom; it also protects the soft connective tissues of the physical body, which are more vulnerable to repetitive strain injuries. The creativity necessary for choreographing your practice at each of these three levels and bringing them all together seamlessly comes through consistent study and time spent testing ideas between practice sessions. Through such practice, you will discover how the shapes of certain poses fit together when transitioning to other poses, as well as the synchronization and coordination of movement and breath at any level of intensity using a continuous stream of breath without disturbance.

## PRACTICE CHOREOGRAPHY

In the course of establishing a personal yoga practice, it is important to experience how the different styles of practice affect us physically and psychologically. As we gain more experience and knowledge, we all tend to develop biases toward styles of practice we like and against those we dislike. One of the most helpful—but irritating—things I heard often as a beginner was "Don't get attached to your likes and dislikes." Essentially, "Practice what you don't like most days and occasionally practice what you do like."

In addition to bias, there are other, subtler influences on your decisions when contemplating a way to practice. The time of day, the weather, the season, your constitution, your disposition, your age, the phase of the moon, your health, your menstrual cycle, menopause, pregnancy, and no doubt more, influence how you choose or create your practices. To grow creatively, you learn (mostly through trial and error) how to adapt or modify certain aspects of your practice from the knowledge and experience you have accumulated so far in order to address what shows up each day on your mat. If you don't, your practice is likely to aggravate imbalances and produce ill-desired effects.

### Styles of Practice

After decades of personal exploration and observation of various teachings of *hatha* yoga, it appears to me that most of today's yoga can be placed into three distinct styles of practice, or a combination thereof: static, dynamic, and restorative. The first two also have subcategories, as follows:

- **STATIC** uses extended holds of the poses to build strength, stamina, and flexibility.
    1. *ha* (masculine principles): endurance, power, active, strength, heating
    2. *tha* (feminine principles): sensitivity, fluid, passive, contemplative, cooling

- **DYNAMIC** incorporates flowing transitions between poses with short holds to build grace, lightness, and balance.
    1. *ha* (masculine principles): linear, fast, agility, heating
    2. *tha* (feminine principles): spontaneous, slow, creative, cooling

- **RESTORATIVE** is therapeutic and uses props with extended holds in passive, supported poses to help balance and reset biomechanical and neurological processes in the body and central nervous system.

## Composition of Sequences

If you want to know whether your yoga practice is serving you, look at your relationships . . . see if you're becoming kinder to yourself and those in your life.
**Shandor Remete**

I've experienced and enjoyed many different practices of physical yoga around the world, learning from a number of the top international teachers in the East and West. All of them taught me a variety of practices that helped me understand more about yoga and myself. I have memorized many of the sequences they taught me, as well as many of the intricate physical details for activating muscular effort and physical alignment in hundreds of poses; I have attended numerous advanced trainings, workshops, and teacher intensives; and I have read hundreds of yoga books by authors famous and less well known. But none of what I learned or received from any teacher taught me how to develop a truly personal practice. After twenty-five years of practicing yoga, I was still unclear how to think for myself when I stepped onto the mat, how to respond to what showed up each day, or how to design an efficient practice that created mental and physical balance in life for myself and the students who were showing up in my classes.

Then one day it became a little clearer to me: all the circumstances of my life and the path I had taken had provided me with everything I needed. I had longed for and sought out simplicity, balance, and contentment in every aspect of my life. I remembered experiences both on and off the mat when I had felt these things the most, and I began to compile my ideas, eliminating anything that my intuition indicated was unnecessary or untrue. I had learned so much, but I had to get rid of most of what I had "collected." What evolved were the three Practice Principles. Over time I realized that these principles also created a context of understanding and awareness that could apply in my life and others' lives.

The Practice Principles provide suggestions on how to change the way you relate to movement, using the physical and subtle body forces of gravity and grace. Applying these principles helps you discover what works to creatively sustain and deepen your personal practice over extended periods and through different phases of life. Over the past decade, *no practice I have done or taught has been the same*. As long as you maintain a commitment to respond creatively to whatever arrives with you when stepping onto your mat, the sequences and the poses that emerge from you will continually evolve. Since I created them ten years ago, the Practice Principles have remained mostly unchanged. They are still applicable to what I practice and what I teach, from basic beginner-level classes to more advanced, intermediate-level classes. For the beginner, I recommend working patiently toward the mastery of these principles and respecting the limitations experienced with each practice. For the intermediate student, I recommend diligently discarding all that is not serving you in your practice and reminding yourself of the passionate curiosity you possessed when you were a beginner.

Do only what is possible for each day and skip the rest. Go further if there is an invitation coming from your own inner wisdom to do so. This effort will bear fruit as long as you consistently embrace your relationship to your practice and the things that arise in it, and as long as you aspire to balance.

## BASIC STRUCTURE OF PRACTICE SEQUENCES

Although the poses within the practice sequences have varied over time, the basic structure has remained the same and is grouped into three parts: opening, dynamic, and closing.

- **OPENING SEQUENCE:** This sequence contains preliminary exercises for creating space in all the major joints in the body in preparation for the practice of yoga *asana*. It also stimulates subtle energy points (*marmas*) in the body, which in turn stimulate channels of subtle energy responsible for circulation, respiration, elimination, flexibility, removing sluggishness, balancing blood pressure, and building mental focus and clarity. This work is done mostly on the floor in a slow, mindful series that includes both stretching and strengthening exercises. The challenge in this work is to touch whatever physical or mental limitation or discomfort that arises, as softly as you can, without excessive muscular force, while also maintaining a present-moment awareness with your breath—its rhythm, its sound, and its texture. Your own creativity is encouraged at times when, due to a current or preexisting condition (like an injury), you feel the need to adapt poses that you are not capable of during your practice, using props if needed to stay in a pose at the level that works best for you. Within the practices of the opening sequence are many of the subtle body "seeds" of attention for the more advanced poses found in the dynamic and closing sequences.

- **DYNAMIC SEQUENCE:** This sequence has been created to build heat in the body and increase life force by strengthening the core energies responsible for digestion. These exercises, which are done mostly standing on the feet or the hands, are designed to stretch and strengthen the legs and arms, soften and tone the abdomen, increase the capacity of the lungs, and improve cardiovascular circulation and elimination. You are encouraged to do only what you are capable of doing and to never force things that you can't do. For more accomplished practitioners, introduce creative variations that give you a deeper experience to meet those places in your body that present challenges, physical or psychological.

- **CLOSING SEQUENCE:** Finally, this sequence is responsible for cooling and quieting the nervous system and refining the quality of stillness in your body that resulted from your practice, mentally and physically. These exercises are mostly floor poses and inversions, the latter of which reverse gravity through the internal organs and increase circulation to the spine and cranial/sacral channels. This work transitions your effort from the active to the passive in preparation for meditation.

Using this structure to compose your practice and integrating the Practice Principles will help you enjoy the next step of the journey you have embarked on, one that will take you in the direction of a truly personal practice. The work along this path develops a sensitivity to the inner teacher of body sensations, empowering you to confidently decide how to practice each day. It will help you avoid the obstacle of boredom in following a set routine and stimulate your own creative force to keep the mind focused in the present moment. This is where you are able to explore and observe the subtle spaces and feelings in the body that are connected—and discover those that are disconnected. Through the wisdom of your own experience, you will naturally reconnect and restore balance to yourself.

> First in the mind,
> then in the body.
> The abdomen relaxes,
> then the breath sinks into the bones.
> The life force is relaxed
> and the body calm.
> It is always in the mind.
> Being able to breathe properly
> leads to agility.
> The softest
> will then become
> the strongest.
>
> Wu Yu-hsiang

When the student is ready, the teacher
will appear. When the student is truly
ready . . . the teacher will disappear.

**Unknown**

# *Afterword*

## *Steps from Here*

The desire to learn more has led me to this point in my understanding, although exactly how I arrived here is no clearer to me after all these years. It is, and seems that it will always be, such a mystery—an example of profound grace. Even so, I trust it, as I do gravity, the invisible force we live with that keeps us grounded physically and psychologically. And from some deep knowing, I feel grace is also the natural order of things, which works in a paradoxical way when surrender is present, when we release expectations and recognize the beauty in things as they are, in any given moment, in the world as it is. This is what my practice has taught me, and I hope it will inspire you to appreciate what yoga uncovers within your practice and to feel genuinely grateful for this process that offers us the ability to return, day after day, to an understanding and awareness of our true nature and the nature we all dwell in.

# Acknowledgments

First and foremost, I extend heartfelt thanks to Tawny Sterios, my guru of patience, kindness, understanding, and love. To Athena Sterios, my guru of play, laughter, joy, forgiveness (for the sacrifices you made while I wrote) and for overcoming the fear of being tickled.

To my parents, I share my deep gratitude for everything you provided me, in ways I will never fully understand. I am in awe of the sacrifices you made to create an abundant life for three young boys growing up.

To Shandor Remete, for introducing me to the true potential of *hatha* yoga and guiding me through illusions and the appearances of darkness. To Father Charlie Moore, for inspiring me to see the world through a different set of lenses and introducing me to gravity, grace, and levity and the idea that ecstasy is the prime mover of all species.

To Dr. Richard Moss, for introducing me to the true meaning of softness and presence. To James Bailey, for simultaneous gentleness, strength, and brotherhood and for guidance with your powerful intellect at just the right moments.

To Eoin Finn, for your masterful example of teaching with humor, passion, and connection. To Fiji McAlpine, my guru of calm, for modeling how to manage parenthood, marriage, and life as a busy yogini. To Tiffany Cruikshank, for sharing your insights and discoveries of recent scientific research on connective tissue. To Mary Prefontaine, for generosity of spirit and impeccable timing "on the homestretch" and the hospitality of your amazing beachfront writer's retreat to complete this book.

To the founders, staff, and community of Esalen Institute, for supporting my learning and teaching over so many years and for the opportunity to be a part of your extraordinary vision.

And finally to Sheridan McCarthy, for inspiration, motivation, and your exquisite editing to bring all of my writing together into a beautiful *and concise* reflection of the life I have lived on and off my mat for the past forty-five years.

# Appendix

## Subtle Body Guidesheets

The Subtle Body Guidesheets that follow provide a quick and simple tool for seeing the inner workings of a pose holistically, physically, and energetically: how basic components of the subtle body operate individually or together as a whole. Presenting this information graphically helps avoid the shortcomings of a left-brain, linear approach to understanding that comes when reading a book or listening to verbal instruction from a teacher; it allows access to the right-brain intelligence that comes with a "whole picture" perspective, helping you think intuitively, creatively, personally, and universally. With familiarity, seeing *hatha* yoga presented this way will instantly give you a sense of a pose "below the skin," with opportunities to discover for yourself the hidden aspects and nuances your experiences bring to learning.

Graphical symbols on each guidesheet are used to identify components or actions found in the physical and subtle bodies for each pose. To help you translate what the symbols represent, the symbols legend index gives a detailed description for each. What is included forms a basic short list of elements to recognize and incorporate into the understanding of your practice. The list is by no means definitive or exhaustive and should be considered only as the initial steps toward uncovering what lies within the layers of your unique subtle body.

Also included are guidesheet abbreviations, which are used for frequently applied notes. With use and familiarity, the abbreviations will become like shorthand symbols for common notes as they apply to the drawings.

Guidesheets for the poses described in the Practice Principles section follow:

- Child's Pose (*Balasana*)

- Mountain Pose (*Tadasana*)

- Downward-Facing Dog (*Adho Mukha Svanasana*)

- Standing Backbend (*Utthita Dhanurasana*)

- Seated Straight-Leg Forward Bend (*Paschimottanasana*)

- Standing Side Bend (*Akarasana*)

- Seated Crossed-Leg Twist (*Parivrtta Sukhasana*)

- Headstand (*Sirsasana*)

Online at LEVITYoGA.com/subtle-body, you can find sample guidesheets for additional beginner-level poses in each of the following categories of poses:

- Seated poses

- Standing poses

- Inversions

- Backbends

- Arm balances

- Prone/supine poses

There are also blank guidesheets (downloadable for free) for you to use and apply what you have learned about the energies of the subtle body described in this section and to uncover for yourself the inner workings of any pose you currently practice at home.

| SYMBOL AND COMPONENT | DESCRIPTION |
|---|---|
| Ground (primary) ▼ | Primary ground for any pose, where body (physical/gross energy and psychological/subtle energy) meets floor; the primary launching pad for subtle body lightness (levity). |
| Ground (secondary) ▽ | Secondary ground for any pose, where any body part rests on the floor without directly influencing the physical or psychological effect of the pose; used more for physical convenience. |
| Attention (inhale/subtle expansion) ○ | Where your attention is placed on the inhale, to feel (or visualize) the subtle expansion and coolness of the breath; where your mind is, the breath follows, and a feeling of pause/calm appears. |
| Attention (exhale/subtle release) • | Where your attention is placed on the exhale, to feel (or visualize) the subtle release and warmth of the breath; where your mind is, the breath retreats, softness takes its place, a feeling of space opens, intuitive response appears. |
| Attention (both cycles) ◉ | When your attention is in the same place for both the inhale and the exhale. |
| *Drishti* ◖ | Location of focused visual attention for the outer gaze, eyes open (OG) or inner gaze, eyes closed (IG). |
| Line of Energy (active/direct) → | Direct, physical/muscular effort initiated by intuitive response to softness or release of subconscious tension, usually on the exhale. |
| Line of Energy (passive/indirect) ⇢ | Indirect, gravity-supplied movement or subtle body sensation initiated by intuitive response to softness or release of subconscious tension, usually on the exhale. |

**FIGURE 17**  Symbols legend index

| SYMBOL AND COMPONENT | DESCRIPTION |
|---|---|
| Extension (active)<br>⟷ | *Extension in the spine*, when either one or both end(s) are actively extended through physical/muscular effort, usually on the exhale; *in the limbs* (arms and legs), when the ends (hands and feet) are actively extended through physical/muscular effort, usually on the exhale. |
| Extension (passive)<br>◄--► | *Extension in the spine*, when both ends are passively extended by gravity-supplied movement or subtle body sensation of softness and release of subconscious tension, usually on an exhale; *in the limbs* (arms and legs), when the ends (hands and feet) are passively extended through physical/muscular effort, usually on the exhale. |
| Contraction (active)<br>→← | *Contraction in the torso and limbs*, when muscles contract actively, from mentally imposed effort for additional pose support, or movement further into a pose on an inhale, exhale, or both. |
| Contraction (passive)<br>--►◄-- | *Contraction in the torso and limbs*, when muscles contract passively, from a natural, gravitational response for additional pose support or movement further into a pose on an inhale, exhale, or both. |
| External Rotation (active)<br>↷ | Mentally imposed muscular turning of a limb about its axis of rotation *away* from the midline of the body (lateral). |
| External Rotation (passive)<br>⤻ | Gravity-initiated turning of a limb about its axis of rotation *away* from the midline of the body (lateral). |
| Internal Rotation (active)<br>⌃ | Mentally imposed muscular turning of a limb about its axis of rotation *toward* the midline of the body (medial). |
| Internal Rotation (passive)<br>⌃ | Gravity-initiated muscular turning of a limb about its axis of rotation *toward* the midline of the body (medial). |

**FIGURE 17**   Symbols legend index (*cont.*)

| | | | |
|---|---|---|---|
| AM | Abdominal Muscles | IE | Inner Ear |
| AO | Abdominal Organs | IG | Inner Gaze |
| BB | Back-Body | IPS | Iliopsoas |
| BOS | Back of Skull | NVL | Navel |
| BOT | Back of Throat | OG | Outer Gaze |
| BT | Brain Tissue | OM | Optic Muscles |
| CB | Collarbone | PB | Pubic Bone |
| CM | Calf Muscles | PF | Pelvic Floor |
| COG | Center of Gravity | PSM | Paraspinal Muscles |
| COM | Corners of Mouth | QM | Quadricep Muscles |
| DPH | Diaphragm | ROT | Root of Tongue |
| EB | Eyeballs | SB | Sitting Bones |
| FHD | Forehead | SBN | Skin Below Navel |
| FLB | Frontal Lobe of Brain | SM | Sphincter Muscles (urinary & anal) |
| FOT | Front of Throat | SOT | Sides of Tongue |
| FSB | Front, Side & Back (of lungs) | TB | Tailbone |
| GM | Gluteal Muscles | TG | Thyroid Gland |
| GRN | Groin | TOC | Tip of Chin |
| HC | Hip Crease (upper thigh at hip) | TOL | Top of Lung |
| HOJ | Hinge of Jaw | TOM | Texture of Mat |
| HRT | Heart | UL | Upper Lung |
| HSM | Hamstring Muscles | | |

**FIGURE 18** Guidesheet abbreviations

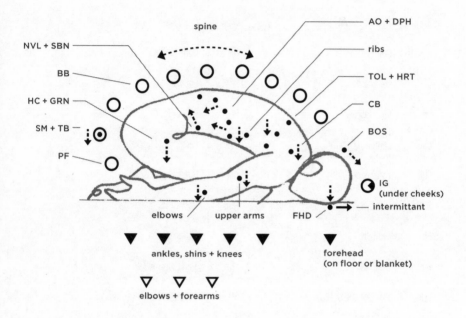

**spine**

**NVL + SBN**

**BB**

**HC + GRN**

**SM + TB**

**PF**

**AO + DPH**

**ribs**

**TOL + HRT**

**CB**

**BOS**

**IG**
(under cheeks)

**intermittant**

**elbows**   **upper arms**   **FHD**

**ankles, shins + knees**

**forehead**
(on floor or blanket)

**elbows + forearms**

**SUBTLE BODY GUIDESHEET 1**   Child's Pose (*Balasana*)

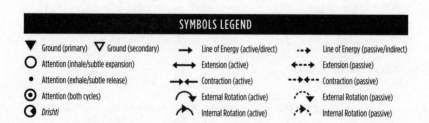

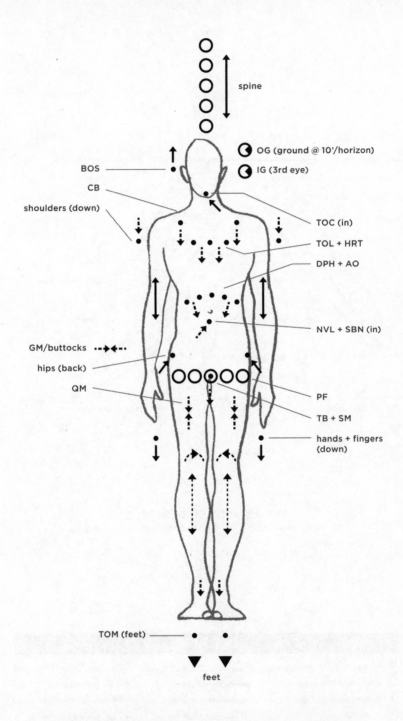

spine

OG (ground @ 10'/horizon)

IG (3rd eye)

BOS

CB

shoulders (down)

TOC (in)

TOL + HRT

DPH + AO

NVL + SBN (in)

GM/buttocks

hips (back)

QM

PF

TB + SM

hands + fingers (down)

TOM (feet)

feet

**SUBTLE BODY GUIDESHEET 2**   Mountain Pose (*Tadasana*)

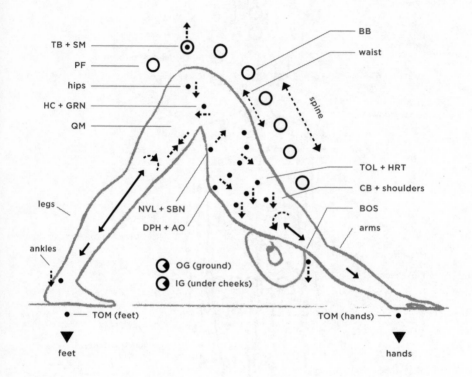

**SUBTLE BODY GUIDESHEET 3**
Downward-Facing Dog (*Adho Mukha Svanasana*)

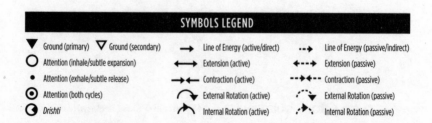

**SYMBOLS LEGEND**

| ▼ Ground (primary) | ▽ Ground (secondary) | → Line of Energy (active/direct) | ⇢ Line of Energy (passive/indirect) |
|---|---|---|---|
| ○ Attention (inhale/subtle expansion) | | ↔ Extension (active) | ⬸⇢ Extension (passive) |
| • Attention (exhale/subtle release) | | →← Contraction (active) | ⇢⇠ Contraction (passive) |
| ◉ Attention (both cycles) | | ↻ External Rotation (active) | ↺ External Rotation (passive) |
| ◖ *Drishti* | | ↶ Internal Rotation (active) | ↷ Internal Rotation (passive) |

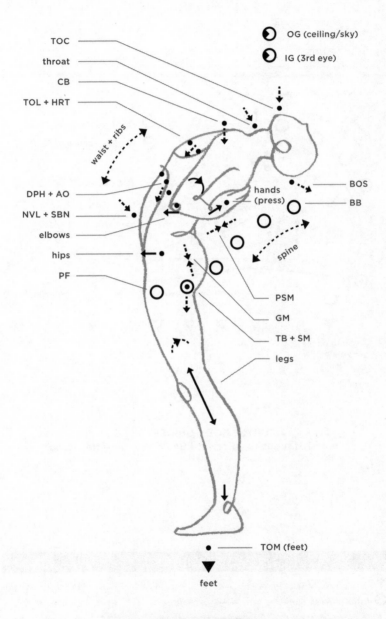

**SUBTLE BODY GUIDESHEET 4**
Standing Backbend (*Utthita Dhanurasana*)

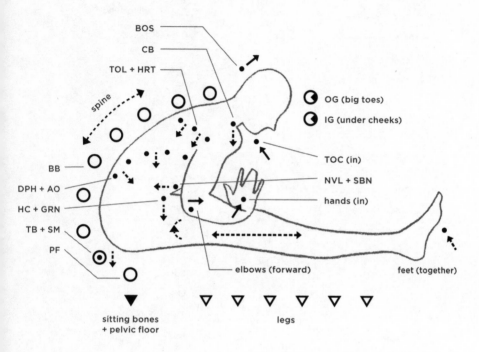

BOS
CB
TOL + HRT

spine

OG (big toes)
IG (under cheeks)

TOC (in)
NVL + SBN
hands (in)

BB
DPH + AO
HC + GRN
TB + SM
PF

elbows (forward)

feet (together)

sitting bones
+ pelvic floor

legs

**SUBTLE BODY GUIDESHEET 5**
Seated Straight-Leg Forward Bend (*Paschimottanasana*)

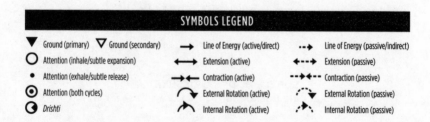

| SYMBOLS LEGEND | | |
|---|---|---|
| ▼ Ground (primary)   ▽ Ground (secondary) | → Line of Energy (active/direct) | ⋯▶ Line of Energy (passive/indirect) |
| ◯ Attention (inhale/subtle expansion) | ◀——▶ Extension (active) | ◀--▶ Extension (passive) |
| • Attention (exhale/subtle release) | →▶◀— Contraction (active) | --▶◀-- Contraction (passive) |
| ◉ Attention (both cycles) | ↷ External Rotation (active) | ⤸ External Rotation (passive) |
| ◖ *Drishti* | ⤴ Internal Rotation (active) | ⤏ Internal Rotation (passive) |

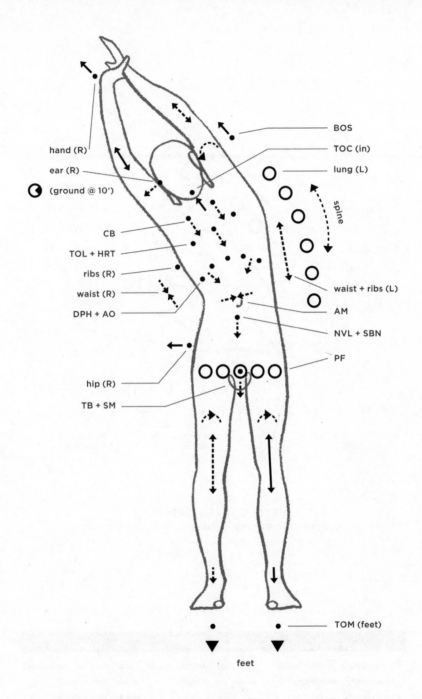

**SUBTLE BODY GUIDESHEET 6** Standing Side Bend (*Akarasana*)

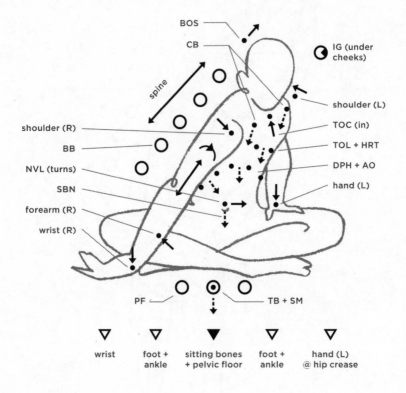

**SUBTLE BODY GUIDESHEET 7**
Seated Crossed-Leg Twist (*Parivrtta Sukhasana*)

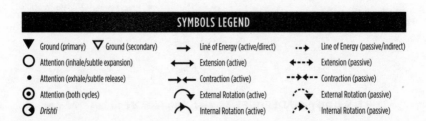

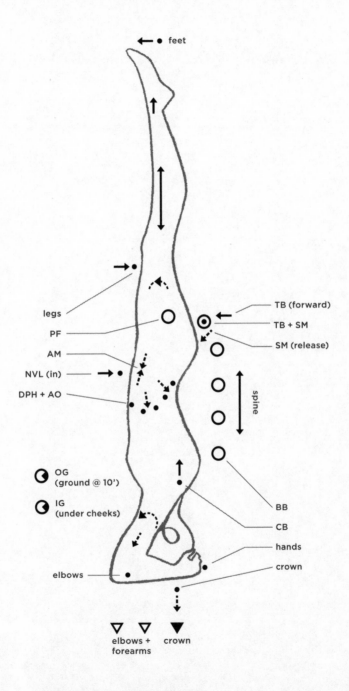

feet

TB (forward)

TB + SM

SM (release)

legs

PF

AM

NVL (in)

DPH + AO

spine

OG
(ground @ 10')

IG
(under cheeks)

BB

CB

hands

crown

elbows

▽ ▽ ▼
elbows + crown
forearms

**SUBTLE BODY GUIDESHEET 8** Headstand (*Sirsasana*)

# Notes

1. Jane Roberts, *Oversoul Seven and the Museum of Time* (Englewood Cliffs, NJ: Prentice Hall, 1984), 49.
2. "Evolution of Consciousness, Grace, Gravity, Love: Father Charles Moore," discussion between Charles Moore and Robert Muller, filmed circa 2006, YouTube video, 6:45, published by KnewWays, August 13, 2009, youtube.com/watch?v=il5SgU_AzNE.
3. Glenn Geffcken, "Lightness of Heart," *Heart and Mind* (blog), Balanced Is, October 13, 2014, balancedis.com/2014/10/lightness-of-heart.
4. Elizabeth H. Page, "Structure and Function of the Skin," *Merck Manual Consumer Version*, updated February 2017, merckmanuals.com/home /skin-disorders/biology-of-the-skin/structure-and-function-of-the-skin.
5. Esther P. Gardner, "Touch," in *Encyclopedia of Life Sciences* (New York: John Wiley and Sons, 2001), 10.
6. Gardner, "Touch," 8.
7. Laurent Misery, "Neuro-Immuno-Cutaneous System (NICS)," *Pathologie-Biologie* 44, no. 10 (December 1996): 867–74, ncbi.nlm .nih.gov/pubmed/9157366.
8. Misery, "Neuro-Immuno-Cutaneous System (NICS)."
9. "Psychogalvanic Reflex," *Encyclopedia Britannica*, updated July 28, 2017, britannica.com/science/psychogalvanic-reflex.
10. "Sense of Touch," *Home Science Tools*, learning-center.homesciencetools .com/article/skin-touch.
11. Sandra Blakeslee and Matthew Blakeslee, *The Body Has a Mind of Its Own: How Body Maps in Your Brain Help You Do (Almost) Everything Better* (New York: Random House, 2007), 8–14.
12. Bruce Lipton, *The Biology of Belief: Unleashing the Power of Consciousness, Matter, and Miracles* (Carlsbad, CA: Hay House, 2008).
13. Robert Schleip, et al., "The Bodywide Fascial Network as a Sensory Organ for Haptic Perception," *Journal of Motor Behavior* 46, no. 3 (2014): 191–92; P. G. Pvana, et al., "Painful Connections: Densification Versus Fibrosis of Fascia," *Current Pain and Headache Reports* 18, no. 441 (2014): 2–3, dx.doi.org/10.1007/s11916-014 -0441-4; S. C. Gandevia, "Proprioception, Tensegrity, and Motor Control," *Journal of Motor Behavior*, 46, no. 3 (2014): 200;

M. T. Turvey and S. T. Fonseca, "The Medium of Haptic Perception: A Tensegrity Hypothesis," *Journal of Motor Behavior*, 46 (2014): 143–87.

14. Robert Schleip, "Mechanotransduction: From the Cellular Level to the Whole Body," in *Textbook of Osteopathic Medicine*, ed. Johannes Mayer and Clive Standen (Munich: Elsevier, 2017), 120–22.

15. Ed Colgate, "Haptic Perception: A Primer," *Feeling Disruptive* (blog), Medium.com, September 25, 2016, medium.com/feelingdisruptive /haptic-perception-a-primer-8c46efb0919d.

16. Michael T. Turvey and Sérgio T. Fonseca, "The Medium of Haptic Perception: A Tensegrity Hypothesis," *Journal of Motor Behavior* 46, no. 3 (2014): 145, ncbi.nlm.nih.gov/pubmed/24628057.

17. Blakeslee and Blakeslee, *Body Has a Mind of Its Own*, 163–69.

18. Blakeslee and Blakeslee, 61–62.

19. "Persistence Hunting," Wikipedia, October 1, 2018, en.wikipedia.org /wiki/Persistence_hunting.

20. Christopher McDougall, *Born to Run: A Hidden Tribe, Superathletes, and the Greatest Race the World Has Never Seen* (New York: Vintage, 2011).

21. McDougall, *Born to Run*, 156.

22. McDougall, 177.

23. Karlfried Graf Dürckheim, *Hara: The Vital Center of Man* (Rochester, VT: Inner Traditions, 2004).

24. John E. Hall, *Guyton and Hall Textbook of Medical Physiology*, 12th ed. (Philadelphia: Saunders Elsevier, 2011), 755.

25. "Dopamine," Wikipedia, updated November 21, 2018, en.wikipedia .org/wiki/Dopamine.

26. "Serotonin," Wikipedia, updated November 10, 2018, en.wikipedia .org/wiki/Serotonin.

27. Behtash Ghazi Nezami and Shanthi Srinivasan, "Enteric Nervous System in the Small Intestine: Pathophysiology and Clinical Implications," *Current Gastroenterology Reports* 12, no. 5 (October 2010): 358–65.

28. Adam Hadhazy, "Think Twice: How the Gut's 'Second Brain' Influences Mood and Well-Being," *Scientific American*, February 12, 2010, scientificamerican.com/article/gut-second-brain.

29. "The Top 10 Causes of Death," World Health Organization, May 24, 2018, who.int/en/news-room/fact-sheets/detail /the-top-10-causes-of-death.

30. Paul P. Pearsall, *The Heart's Code: Tapping the Wisdom and Power of Our Heart Energy* (New York: Harmony, 1998), 13.

31. Pearsall, *Heart's Code*, 4–5.

32. Pearsall, 39.

33. Pearsall, 42–43.

34. Pearsall, 25.

35. Pearsall, 45–50.

36. Paraphrased and directly quoted from Vasant Lad, *Marma Points of Ayurveda: The Energy Pathways for Healing Body, Mind, and Consciousness with a Comparison to Traditional Chinese Medicine* (Albuquerque, NM: Ayurvedic Press, 2015), 241.

37. Charles Moore, *Synthesis Remembered: Awakening Original Innocence* (Soquel, CA: Mooredune Publications, 2006), 9.

38. Lipton, *Biology of Belief*, 102.

39. Lipton, xv.

40. Lipton, x.

41. Lipton, 60–61.

42. Lipton, 80–81. Studies cited by Lipton include C. W. F. McClare, "Resonance in Bioenergetics," *Annals of the New York Academy of Sciences* 227 (1974): 74–97; Klaus Schulten, "Electron Transfer: Exploiting Thermal Motion," *Science* 290, no. 5489 (2000): 61–62; M. Chergui, "Controlling Biological Functions," *Science* 313, no. 5791 (2006): 1246–47; and Susan Gaidos and Nicolle Rager Fuller, "Living Physics: From Green Leaves to Bird Brains, Biological Systems May Exploit Quantum Phenomena," *Science News* 175, no. 10 (2009): 26–29.

43. Lipton, 102.

44. Lipton, 102.

45. Lipton, 102.

46. Lipton, 103.

47. Lipton, 98.

48. Lipton, 133.

49. Belleruth Naparstek, *Your Sixth Sense: Unlocking the Power of Your Intuition* (New York: HarperOne, 1997), 40.

50. Naparstek, *Your Sixth Sense*, 106–10.

51. Naparstek, 109; Lipton, *Biology of Belief*, 134; Cheyenne Diaz, "The Marvelous Properties of Gamma Brain Waves," *Mindvalley* (blog), January 2018, blog.mindvalley.com/gamma-brain-waves.

52. Diaz, "Marvelous Properties of Gamma Brain Waves"; Naparstek, *Your Sixth Sense*.

53. Naparstek, 107.

54. Naparstek, 71–72.

55. Naparstek, 103

56. Naparstek, 103–4.

57. Itzhak Bentov, *Stalking the Wild Pendulum: On the Mechanics of Consciousness* (Rochester, VT: Inner Traditions/Bear & Company, 1977), 86–87.

58. Naparstek, *Your Sixth Sense*, 104.

59. Naparstek, 110.

60. Steven Kotler, "Flow States and Creativity," *Psychology Today*, February 25, 2014, psychologytoday.com/us/blog/the-playing-field/201402 /flow-states-and-creativity.

61. Melissa Conrad Stoppler, "Endorphins: Natural Pain and Stress Fighters," MedicineNet, June 13, 2018, medicinenet.com/script /main/art.asp?articlekey=55001.

62. James McIntosh, "What Is Serotonin and What Does It Do?" *Medical News Today*, February 2, 2018, medicalnewstoday.com/kc /serotonin-facts-232248.

63. Naparstek, *Your Sixth Sense*, 49.

64. Naparstek, 71.

65. Naparstek, 76.

66. Thomas Reid, *Essays on the Active Powers of the Human Mind*, ed. B. A. Brody (Cambridge, MA: MIT Press, 1969; Glasgow, UK: R. Griffin and Co., 1843).

67. Naparstek, *Your Sixth Sense*, 82.

68. Naparstek, 76.

69. Naparstek, 43.

70. Quoted in Naparstek, *Your Sixth Sense*, 106–7.

71. Naparstek, *Your Sixth Sense*.

72. Naparstek, 108.

73. Naparstek, 101.

74. "Itzhak Bentov," Wikipedia, updated September 5, 2018, en.wikipedia.org/wiki/Itzhak_Bentov#cite_note-secrets-3.

75. Bentov, *Stalking the Wild Pendulum*, 122.

76. Pearsall, *Heart's Code*, 194.

77. Pearsall, 194.

78. James Gleick, *Chaos: Making a New Science* (New York: Penguin Books, 1988).

79. Pearsall, *Heart's Code*, 198

80. Pearsall, 204–6.

81. Norman Cousins, *Head First: The Biology of Hope* (New York: E. P. Dutton, 1989).

82. Pearsall, *Heart's Code*, 197.

83. S. N. Goenka and William Hart, *The Art of Living* (Igatpuri, Maharashtra, India: Vipassana Research Institute, 1988), 25–26.

84. Hareesh [Christopher Wallis], "The Real Story on the Chakras," Hareesh.org, February 5, 2016, hareesh.org/blog/2016/2/5 /the-real-story-on-the-chakras.

85. Hareesh, "The Real Story."

86. Hareesh [Christopher Wallis], "The Power of Subtle Impressions (Samskaara Theory)," Hareesh.org, October 6, 2015, hareesh.org /blog/2015/9/21/impressions-of-past-lives.

87. Hareesh, "The Power."

88. Hareesh.

89. Harish Johari, *Chakras: Energy Centers of Transformation* (Rochester, VT: Destiny Books, 2000), 1–2.

90. Michael Roach and Christie McNally, *The Essential Yoga Sutra: Ancient Wisdom for Your Yoga* (New York: Doubleday, 2000).

91. Roach and McNally, *Essential Yoga Sutra*, 77.

92. Roach and McNally, 78.

93. Roach and McNally, 79

94. Roach and McNally, 80.

95. Shandor Remete, *Shadow Yoga, Chaya Yoga: The Principles of Hatha Yoga* (Berkeley, CA: North Atlantic, 2010), 56–57.

96. Roach and McNally, *Essential Yoga Sutra*, 81.

97. Michael Roach and Christie McNally, *How Yoga Works* (Wayne, NJ: Diamond Cutter Press, 2005), 108–13.

98. Lad, *Marma Points of Ayurveda*, 52.

99. Swami Digambarji et al., eds., *Vasiṣṭha-Saṃhitā* (Pune, India: Kaivalyadhama S.M.Y.M. Samiti, Lonavla, 1969), 49.

100. This *Yoga Journal* article was published in a now out-of-print issue in 1999. Digital archive version unavailable.

101. Fernando Pagés Ruiz, "Krishnamacharya's Legacy: Modern Yoga's Inventor," *Yoga Journal*, August 28, 2007, yogajournal.com /yoga-101/krishnamacharya-s-legacy.

102. T. K. V. Desikachar with R. H. Cravens, *Health, Healing, and Beyond: Yoga and the Living Tradition of T. Krishnamacharya* (New York: North Point, 1998), 111.

103. Ruiz, "Krishnamacharya's Legacy."

104. Ruiz.

105. Blakeslee and Blakeslee, *Body Has a Mind of Its Own*, 61–62.

106. Loren Fishman, Ellen Saltonstall, and Susan Genis, "Understanding and Preventing Yoga Injuries," *International Journal of Yoga Therapy* 19, no. 1 (2009): 47–53.

107. B. K. S. Iyengar, *Light on Yoga* (New York: Schocken Books, 1979), 189.

# Further Reading

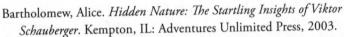

Bartholomew, Alice. *Hidden Nature: The Startling Insights of Viktor Schauberger.* Kempton, IL: Adventures Unlimited Press, 2003.

Bentov, Itzhak. *Stalking the Wild Pendulum: On the Mechanics of Consciousness.* Rochester, VT: Destiny Books, 1988.

Ben-Ze'ev, Aaron. *The Subtlety of Emotions.* Cambridge, MA: MIT Press, 2001.

Blakeslee, Sandra, and Matthew Blakeslee. *The Body Has a Mind of Its Own: How Body Maps in Your Brain Help You Do (Almost) Everything Better.* New York: Random House, 2007.

Chen, Kaiguo, and Zheng Shunchao. *Opening the Dragon Gate: The Making of a Modern Taoist Wizard.* Translated by Thomas Cleary. Tokyo: Charles E. Tuttle, 1996.

Chopra, Deepak. *Life after Death: The Burden of Proof.* New York: Harmony Books, 2006.

Cousins, Norman. *Anatomy of an Illness as Perceived by the Patient: Reflections on Healing and Regeneration.* New York: W. W. Norton, 2005.

Csikszentmihalyi, Mihaly. *Flow: The Psychology of Optimal Experience.* New York: HarperCollins, 1990.

Dale, Cyndi. *The Subtle Body: An Encyclopedia of Your Energetic Anatomy.* Boulder, CO: Sounds True, 2009.

Desikachar, T. K. V., and Richard H. Cravens. *Health, Healing and Beyond: Yoga and the Living Tradition of Krishnamacharya.* New York: North Point, 1998.

Digambarji, Swami, et al. *Vasiṣṭha-Saṃhitā (Yoga Kanda).* Lonavla, Poona, India: Kaivalyadhama S.M.Y.M. Samiti, 1969.

Dürckheim, Karlfried Graf. *Hara: The Vital Center of Man.* Rochester, VT: Inner Traditions, 2004.

Gladwell, Malcolm. *Blink: The Power of Thinking without Thinking.* New York: Little, Brown, 2005.

Goenka, S. N., and William Hart. *The Art of Living.* Igatpuri, Maharashtra, India: Vipassana Research Institute, 1988.

Gottfried, Bob. *Shortcut to Spirituality: Mastering the Art of Inner Peace.* North York, ON: Deeper Dimension, 2004.

Ḥāfiẓ, and Daniel James Ladinsky. *The Gift: Poems.* New York: Penguin, 1999.

Huang, Chungliang Al, and Jerry Lynch. *Thinking Body, Dancing Mind: TaoSports for Extraordinary Performance in Athletics, Business, and Life.* New York: Bantam, 1992.

Iyengar, B. K. S. *Light on Life: The Journey to Wholeness, Inner Peace, and Ultimate Freedom.* Emmaus, PA: Rodale, 2008.

Iyengar, B. K. S. *Yoga: The Path to Holistic Health.* London: Dorling Kindersley, 2001.

Johari, Harish. *Ayurvedic Massage: Traditional Indian Techniques for Balancing Body and Mind.* Rochester, VT: Healing Arts Press, 1996.

Johari, Harish. *Chakras: Energy Centers of Transformation.* Rochester, VT: Destiny Books, 2000.

Kirsch, Irving, Thomas J. Moore, Alan Scoboria, and Sarah S. Nicholls. "The Emperor's New Drugs: An Analysis of Antidepressant Medication Data Submitted to the U.S. Food and Drug Administration." *Prevention & Treatment* 5, no. 1 (2002): dx.doi.org/10.1037/1522-3736.5.1.523a.

Kramer, Joel, and Diana Alstad. *The Guru Papers: Masks of Authoritarian Power.* Berkeley, CA: North Atlantic Books/Frog, 1993.

Kripal, Jeffrey J. *Esalen: America and the Religion of No Religion.* Chicago: University of Chicago Press, 2007.

Krishnamacharya, T. "Salutation to the Teacher and the Eternal One." Unpublished paper distributed to students at the Yoga Mandiram in Madras.

Lad, Vasant, and Anisha Durve. *Marma Points of Ayurveda: The Energy Pathways for Healing Body, Mind, and Consciousness with a Comparison to Traditional Chinese Medicine.* Albuquerque, NM: Ayurvedic Press, 2015.

Lipton, Bruce H. *The Biology of Belief: Unleashing the Power of Consciousness, Matter and Miracles.* Carlsbad, CA: Hay House, 2016.

Lo, Benjamin Pang Jeng, Martin Inn, Susan Foe, and Robert Amacker. *The Essence of T'ai Chi Ch'uan: The Literary Tradition.* Berkeley, CA: North Atlantic Books, 1979.

McDougall, Christopher. *Born to Run: A Hidden Tribe, Superathletes, and the Greatest Race the World Has Never Seen.* New York: Vintage Books, 2011.

Moore, Charles L. *Synthesis Remembered: Awakening Original Innocence.* Soquel, CA: Mooredune Publications, 2006.

Moss, Richard M. *The Mandala of Being: Discovering the Power of Awareness.* Novato, CA: New World Library, 2007.

Moss, Richard M. *The Second Miracle: Intimacy, Spirituality, and Conscious Relationships*. Berkeley, CA: Celestial Arts, 1995.

Myers, Thomas, and James Earls. *Fascial Release of Structural Balance*. Berkeley: North Atlantic Books, 2017.

Naparstek, Belleruth. *Your Sixth Sense: Activating Your Psychic Potential*. New York: HarperOne, 1997.

Pearsall, Paul P. *The Heart's Code: Tapping the Wisdom and Power of Our Heart Energy*. New York: Broadway Books, 1999.

Pert, Candace B. *Molecules of Emotion*. New York: Pocket Books, 1997.

Remete, Shandor. *Shadow Yoga: Chaya Yoga*. Berkeley, CA: North Atlantic, 2006.

Rieker, Hans-Ulrich, and Elsy Becherer. *The Yoga of Light: The Classic Esoteric Handbook of Kundalini Yoga*. Rochester, VT: Bear & Company, 1997.

Roach, Michael, and Christie McNally. *The Essential Yoga Sutra: A New Translation and Commentary of Patanjali's Ancient Classic*. New York: Doubleday, 2005.

Roach, Michael, and Christie McNally. *How Yoga Works: Healing Yourself and Others with the Yoga Sutra*. Wayne, NJ: Diamond Cutter Press, 2005.

Saraswati, Muktibodhananda, and Satyananda Saraswati. *Swara Yoga: The Tantric Science of Brain Breathing*. Munger, Bihar, India: Bihar School of Yoga, 1984.

Satchidananda, Sri Swami. *The Yoga Sūtras of Patañjali*. Buckingham, VA: Integral Yoga Publications, 2012.

Sears, J. P. *How to Be Ultra Spiritual: 12½ Steps to Spiritual Superiority*. Boulder, CO: Sounds True, 2017.

*The Taittirîya Upanishad, with the Commentaries of Sankarâchârya, Suresvarâcharya and Sâyana (Vidyâranya)*. Translated by A. Mahadeva Sastri. Mysore, India: G.T.A. Printing Press, 1903.

Taylor, Jill Bolte. *My Stroke of Insight: A Brain Scientist's Personal Journey*. New York: Viking, 2008.

Tiller, William A. *Science and Human Transformation: Subtle Energies, Intentionality, and Consciousness*. Walnut Creek, CA: Pavior Publications, 1997.

Todd, Mabel Elsworth. *The Thinking Body: A Study of the Balancing Forces of Dynamic Man*. New York: Dance Horizons, 1968.

Walker, Lauren. *Energy Medicine Yoga: Amplify the Healing Power of Your Yoga Practice*. Boulder, CO: Sounds True, 2014.

Weil, Simone. *Gravity and Grace*. New York: Routledge, 2002.

Whitman, Walt. *Song of Myself: The First and Final Editions of the Great American Poem*. American Renaissance Books. 2010. Kindle edition.

Whitman, Walt, and Lawrence Clark Powell. *Leaves of Grass: Poems of Walt Whitman*. New York: T. Y. Crowell, 1986.

Zarrilli, Philip B. *When the Body Becomes All Eyes: Paradigms, Discourses, and Practices of Power in Kalarippayattu, a South Indian Martial Art*. Oxford: Oxford University Press, 2001.

# About the Author

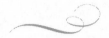

Peter Sterios has been part of the global yoga community for over four decades as a teacher, writer, designer, and entrepreneur based in San Luis Obispo, California. He is the founder of Manduka® and LEVITYoGA™ and a former contributing editor for *Yoga Journal*. Peter's first yoga instructional DVD, *Gravity & Grace: Yoga for Finding Your Inner Teacher*, was selected in *Yoga Journal*'s "top 15 yoga videos of all time," and his unique online classes are featured at YogaAnytime.com. Peter also cofounded karmaNICA™, a charitable organization supporting impoverished school children in western Nicaragua. For three years, Peter taught yoga at the White House for one of Michelle Obama's anti-obesity initiatives (2011–2013), and in 2018, he was invited to the Pentagon to share ideas about the therapeutic effects of yoga for the US Marine Corps. For more information about Peter's lighthearted approach to and insights about the evolving art of yoga, visit LEVITYoGA.com.

# About Sounds True

Sounds True is a multimedia publisher whose mission is to inspire and support personal transformation and spiritual awakening. Founded in 1985 and located in Boulder, Colorado, we work with many of the leading spiritual teachers, thinkers, healers, and visionary artists of our time. We strive with every title to preserve the essential "living wisdom" of the author or artist. It is our goal to create products that not only provide information to a reader or listener, but that also embody the quality of a wisdom transmission.

For those seeking genuine transformation, Sounds True is your trusted partner. At SoundsTrue.com you will find a wealth of free resources to support your journey, including exclusive weekly audio interviews, free downloads, interactive learning tools, and other special savings on all our titles.

To learn more, please visit SoundsTrue.com/freegifts or call us toll-free at 800.333.9185.

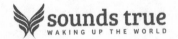

sounds true
WAKING UP THE WORLD